COO 412 674X

COPING WITH A STRESSED NERVOUS SYSTEM

DR KENNETH HAMBLY was educated at The Queen's University of Belfast. He is married with three daughters. After working briefly in Canada, he returned to the UK where he went into general practice. He has always been involved in medical teaching with a particular interest in communication skills, consultation skills and stress management. Dr Hambly has written extensively on these subjects over many years.

ALICE MUIR is an experienced trainer, Chartered Psychologist and Life Coach. She is married with a grown-up family. Alice is the youngest of eight children, and spent her childhood in the Ayrshire countryside, before training at Glasgow and Stirling Universities. She is a member of the British Psychological Society, the General Teaching Council, the International Stress Management Association and the Association for Coaching. Alice has a long-standing interest in personal development, and has been writing and training on the subject, as well as coaching groups and individuals, for the past 25 years.

D1465046

Overcoming Common Problems Series

Selected titles

A full list of titles is available from Sheldon Press,
36 Causton Street, London SW1P 4ST and on our website at
www.sheldonpress.co.uk

Overcoming Common Problems

Coping with a Stressed Nervous System
Autonomic Overload Explained

Dr Kenneth Hambly and Alice Muir

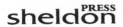

First published in Great Britain in 2005

Sheldon Press
36 Causton Street
London SW1P 4ST

Copyright © Kenneth Hambly and Alice Muir 2005

All rights reserved. No part of this book may be reproduced
or transmitted in any form or by any means,
electronic or mechanical, including photocopying,
recording, or by any information storage and retrieval system,
without permission in writing from the publisher.

The author and publisher have made every effort to
ensure that the external website and email addresses included
in this book are correct and up to date at the time of going
to press. The author and publisher are not responsible for the
content, quality or continuing accessibility of the sites.

British Library Cataloguing-in-Publication Data

A catalogue record for this book is available from the British Library

ISBN 0–85969–946–3

1 3 5 7 9 10 8 6 4 2

Typeset by Deltatype Limited, Birkenhead, Merseyside
Printed in Great Britain by
Ashford Colour Press

**DUNDEE CITY
COUNCIL**

LOCATION
LEISURE READING

ACCESSION NUMBER
C00 412674

SUPPLIER
CAW

PRICE
£7.99

CLASS No.
616.98

DATE
6/12/05

Introduction

This book is about a stress-related condition from which practically no one is immune. We've called it 'stress overload' but it would be more precise to call it *autonomic overload*, or, *autonomic nervous system overload* – when a person becomes unwell because their nervous system just can't cope with all the stimuli it receives on a daily basis. There are plenty of books about stress, but, as far as we know, none on the potentially serious and disabling condition that underlies it, which can affect our entire nervous system and all the workings of our body and mind.

So what is autonomic overload? Autonomic means self-regulating and refers to the part of our nervous system that – usually – more or less looks after itself, governing heart rate, breathing and many other functions of which we are not usually aware. In autonomic overload, our automatic or self-regulating nervous system is overwhelmed by the sheer weight of incoming messages. Perhaps we're dreading a meeting where we have to make a speech, or have a potentially awkward customer to deal with; maybe we have to drive in fast and dangerous traffic; confront a school teacher to talk about an issue with a child; deal with bullying at work. Even meeting friends for a meal out might be a source of stress if, as often happens with stress overload, we end up exhausted before we've even started; or if we're worried that irritable bowel problems will embarrass us. Asking the boss for a favour, getting the kids from school to judo class in time, entertaining our partner's work colleagues – the list is endless, and we're all very familiar with it. This 'chatter' of incoming messages is twenty-first-century life. But, too often, our systems literally cannot cope with it all. We just weren't designed for this level of stimulus. The result: a stressed nervous system that cannot function properly. Physical and psychological symptoms quickly develop, as do changes in the way we behave.

Here are some facts for you to consider:

- Everyone suffers from autonomic overload at some time.
- Autonomic overload makes you ill.
- Autonomic overload in the long term can ruin your life.

1

- Autonomic overload can make you less successful and less happy than you could be.

We all have problems. No one gets a free pass. Life isn't supposed to be easy and for most people it can be very difficult on occasions. Have a look at the following symptoms associated with overload:

- Feeling tired all the time
- Feeling really exhausted
- Waking up feeling tired
- Experiencing pains, often in the neck and shoulders
- Muscle and joint pains
- Headaches
- Terrible head pain like a band round your head
- Pain behind your eyes.
- Stomach upsets such as indigestion, colicky pain and diarrhoea
- A tremor
- A general feeling of shakiness
- Tightness in the chest
- Difficulty getting a breath
- Bladder problems
- Feeling anxious and apprehensive
- Feeling unable to cope
- Having problems concentrating
- Feeling depressed
- Feeling tearful in some situations
- Feeling hopeless much of the time
- Panic attacks
- Avoiding situations you dislike
- Indecision at work or at home
- Anger in inappropriate situations
- Eating or alcohol problems
- Other changes in your usual behaviour
- Lack of assertiveness.

Put like that, it all sounds pretty insurmountable, doesn't it? Yet, we can help you deal with all of these problems. We can also help you deal with your everyday life in a more satisfactory way, even if you have no problems at the moment. That's a promise.

How can we make such a promise? We can do so because all of

the above symptoms are different aspects of the same condition – they are all interrelated. This is the condition we call autonomic overload.

If we help you deal with your autonomic overload, all of your other problems fade away like the early morning mist on a meadow. How do we know we can do that? We know because we have been doing it successfully using the system outlined in this book for many years, and we have had a lifelong interest in the problem.

If you want to feel better and enjoy life more – read on!

1

The Background

explained by Ken Hambly

So, just how can this book help you? We feel we owe you an explanation. I am a doctor, and I have been in practice for 35 years. I began my medical career in hospital obstetrics, but as time went on and my wife and I had more children the decision was made to move to a career in general practice.

This involved spending a year learning what was then the art of family medicine. That meant moving to a small seaside town and dealing directly with the general public, rather than working in a big city teaching hospital. It was quite a change for me, both personally and professionally, as I was used to big clinic situations with plenty of help from nursing staff and support from other more experienced doctors. Now there was just me.

It did not prove to be easy and it soon became clear to me that my time in medical school and in teaching hospital jobs had done little to prepare me for this type of medicine. I was having to learn on the job. I found that I simply had no idea what was wrong with many of my patients who felt unwell and did not know why. I had never heard of or thought about autonomic overload. It was never taught in medical school and hospital doctors didn't understand it.

For some people it was a permanent state, something which made them miserable most of the time. I really felt for these people, an empathy which had roots in my own experience and I did want to help them. Indeed, as a GP in a country town I had an obligation to help them, as there was no one else to whom they could turn, and other doctors I discussed the problem with did not seem to have any answers. There were no clinical psychologists or other psychological workers in general practice when I started, so I was on my own. There are precious few today and waiting lists are huge. I had to start reading and doing the best I could for my patients.

There seemed to be no logic to the problems these patients experienced and I did not know how to treat them. I believe that this is still a problem for young GPs today, but for me it became a source of fascination and interest. There was a reason for this. I recognized in many of my patients echoes of problems I had myself experienced.

All in all, this period was a revelation to me. It seemed as if someone had opened a pair of big barn doors and I could look out on to a new world where everyone had the same kind of problem managing their autonomic overload, but for everyone it was their secret, something they didn't talk about. I was one of them.

The universal truth

There appears to be a sort of conspiracy which holds that everyone is well all the time and can cope with all of life's problems all the time, unless proved ill. People don't ever just 'feel unwell', don't suffer from unpleasant symptoms. You are either ill in a medical sense, or you are fit and well in a medical sense.

Doctors are trained as medical scientists and need to have a close knowledge of the very complex workings of the human body. Like all scientists, they demand proof. If a doctor can't feel something, see something, X-ray or scan something or detect something with a blood test – then the patient is well. Doctors do admit that there's a condition which they call a 'functional illness', just a disorder of normal bodily function, but that diagnosis is a bit of a put-down, almost a suggestion that the patient is malingering. There is also the concept of the 'worried well' about which doctors also talk with a hint of contempt as if such people are 'time wasters'.

Thus the diagnosis is made, but no action is taken. No one is interested in functional disorders and how to treat them. This is the world of the hospital doctor and conventional academic medicine. When a doctor enters general practice, that world is stood on its head.

What the young entrant to family medicine discovers is that major illnesses are rare, but sickness isn't. Many people – I suspect all people – feel ill at some time in their lives and there does not seem to be a medically acceptable reason for the way they feel. It is a universal truth.

One young GP once told me that he was a specialist in managing trivia – perhaps not realizing that what was trivial to him was not necessarily trivial to you, the patient! Some of these undiagnosable problems are catastrophic for an individual, always debilitating and occasionally disabling.

What has gone wrong?

What a strange situation! Here are members of the population sometimes feeling ill, some of us often feeling unwell, and yet we do not feel that we are being treated adequately or even being taken seriously. Is there something wrong with our society's concept of illness? In our society you are either well, or you are ill. There is no 'in between'. Is this an accurate reflection of the true nature of illness, or have we got the definition wrong? I believe that the latter is the case, and I put my 35 years of professional experience on the line here, as well as my personal experience as an individual. The fact is, and this is of fundamental importance to all of us, that 'wellness' is a sliding scale. At one end of that scale and causing many of the problems is autonomic overload.

What is the pathology?

Pathology is what doctors call the scientific cause of an illness, or the tangible nature of the disease process. If you like, it's what can be found at a post-mortem to explain why a person died – never mind that 30 per cent of post-mortems do not demonstrate any pathology. So when you say that you are ill, doctors look for the pathology, the better to treat and cure the illness.

Don't underestimate doctors, they have a heavy and onerous responsibility and it isn't easy. If you have an illness which a doctor can fix, then the doctor has to diagnose it and treat it successfully. You would expect nothing less. Medicine is becoming more and more complex which means that doctors can cure more and more conventional illnesses, often very serious illnesses.

Yet if medically well people get symptoms bad enough to take them to see a doctor, they need help, which they often don't get. They can get reassurance that there is nothing physically wrong with them and that can be of great benefit, but they may not feel much better.

I have known and worked with hundreds of doctors during my professional life, and all that I have worked with have taken their responsibilities very seriously. They aren't all perfect, but then none of us are perfect. By and large, they do their job to the best of their ability. But what is their job? To heal the sick of course, that is what it is and that is what it has been back to the days of Hippocrates. The problem now, in this age of scientific medicine, is just what do we mean by 'the sick'?

Who is ill?

Doctors treat illnesses and find it hard to engage with the concept of 'wellness'. What, then, is illness? Now we are getting into philosophy and metaphysics. Perhaps illness is the state of just 'not feeling well'. If that is the case we have moved from the doctor's definition of illness as being the presence of pathology, either physical or psychological, to the patient's definition – that of disease or just 'not feeling well'. It also raises another problem: if you can't define an illness, if you can't diagnose it and categorize it, how can you make it better? You can't cure something if you don't know what it is. Questions, questions!

Yet this is the key question. A doctor cannot ethically or logically offer treatment of a condition which has not been diagnosed. A doctor can treat symptoms, he or she can treat psychological problems, but there has to be a logic to the treatment because medicine is a science. Doctors actually do the things they are depicted as doing in the TV series *ER* and all the other television medical soaps. Doctors have to think and act logically and ethically, and some day your life may depend upon that fact. I can put it no other way. Other people may have the luxury of trying this and that cure without producing hard evidence that it works, but a doctor cannot miss a crucial diagnosis which might lead to a patient getting the wrong treatment for a serious illness.

Where does this lead?

There is a cord of logic which runs through this discussion, and it was that logic which interested me so many years ago when I first went into general practice. If you remember, I found that I had patients who did not feel well and who had real and disturbing symptoms, but I could not use my medical training to find out why. If because of your experience you agree with me that such distressing symptoms are not 'all in the mind', the logical conclusion has to be that there is another pathology operating.

Take chronic fatigue, for example. I could diagnose appendicitis and even remove a gangrenous appendix, I could manage a breech delivery, I could treat a heart attack, but I could not manage a patient who was tired all the time because of his or her autonomic overload.

The diagnosis of being tired all the time, often abbreviated to 'TATT' or CFS (chronic fatigue syndrome) is very common in medicine and it is used in a rather dismissive way, yet it is of great importance to the person who experiences this overwhelming, crushing, sometimes unmanageable tiredness. The reason why doctors may disregard it is because *it doesn't fit into any medical category*. There are no objective medical tests which will explain it, and so there is no obvious way to treat it. Treatment is pragmatic, and variable.

I have to say that the situation is improving rapidly and doctors now do much better with the types of problem listed in the opening section of this book. But the nature of these illnesses is still not well understood by many and as a result not well treated. Another major problem for doctors is their sheer lack of time. There is also resistance from some patients who believe that there must be something serious wrong with them which some doctor will diagnose and fix, and autonomic overload isn't quite like that.

Stress, the culprit

The main driving force behind autonomic overload is undoubtedly stress. An all too common buzzword, but people who really suffer the autonomic effects of stress do understand its importance, because it makes them ill. It doesn't just make them feel ill, it can make them physically ill. It has been shown that men whose partner suffers from breast cancer have a reduced level of T-cell lymphocytes, the white blood cells that protect us from infection and disease. Furthermore, if an elderly man's wife dies, it has been shown that the man has a reduced longevity compared to others who do not suffer this life event.

So stress is a culprit. That may be work-related stress (WRS), or it might be debt, or problems in the home. It might be divorce or bereavement, but though these life-changing events are demon-strably damaging, they are not the usual cause. More often, it is the slow background stress of a strained relationship, or a bully at work, physical illness, or financial or other relationship problems. Overwork, over-ambitious business goals, pressure from a manager, anything which raises our general level of autonomic arousal will make us more susceptible to the problems it produces.

Stressed people, people with autonomic overload for whatever reason, can be shown to have physical changes which can actually be measured in the laboratory via blood or saliva tests to measure levels of the stress hormone cortisol. If you suffer in this way you are ill. We just have to think about these previously mysterious problems in a different way and perhaps take them more seriously. The treatment of autonomic overload isn't the same as for most other illness, but treatment is needed.

I have suffered from autonomic overload myself in the past. Nothing informs the mind like personal experience. I have experienced many of the symptoms listed in this book. I know what it can be like. I know what it can be like to seek help and not find it. I know what it is like to be disbelieved, or at least not taken seriously. It is possible to be left with severe disturbing symptoms with nowhere to turn, having been told that 'there is nothing wrong with you'. All this adds to the agony of autonomic overload, to the feeling of isolation and reduced confidence. It shouldn't be like that, and it doesn't need to be like that.

How the ideas developed

When I moved to my present practice I contacted Roger Paxton, a clinical psychologist who became interested in my patients and came to my country practice on a weekly basis to offer me advice on how to treat them. We did a little practical research, and developed a way of providing a short course of treatment using verbal advice backed up by handouts. This work was published and it created some interest in the subject. I have used the techniques in different forms in my practice for over twenty-five years. I am eternally grateful to Roger for his help.

Other doctors also developed an interest in dealing with this problem, in particular Dr Richard France and his collaborator who wrote about the use of behaviour therapy techniques in general practice.

THE BACKGROUND

How Alice became involved

Alice Muir, a chartered psychologist with a particular interest and knowledge of this subject, did a research project in my practice. Alice had worked to develop training programmes for use by the general public and was a teacher and lecturer. The research programme was extended to a group of practices and our ideas on how to best manage autonomic overload were crystallized and developed by her until they became much as they are today. We now train nurses and other professionals to treat the condition and help people who suffer from it.

Alice says: 'I first became involved with helping people with nervous overload over twenty years ago now, firstly working with groups, and then working on an individual basis. More recently, I've been able to work with people by post and by e-mail. It has been a fascinating and absorbing twenty years, and I've come into contact with people of all ages, and from all walks of life, all experiencing similar difficulties. Seeking more and more answers to the enigma of nervous overload has led me into areas like managing stress, coping with panic attacks and phobias, confidence-building, life-coaching and assertiveness. This book is an opportunity to share all this with you.'

Your quest – how this book will help

In this book we will explain how autonomic overload causes these problems, and what you can do about it for yourself. Is autonomic overload a medical problem or is it a lifestyle problem, a product of our modern way of living? If the latter, medicalizing it isn't the answer. You need people trained to deal with this problem. But, if you do not have access to such a person – and most of us don't – you can help yourself, but you must go about it the correct way. The treatment methods are straightforward, but most people left to their own devices go about treating themselves the wrong way and end up making themselves worse. That is where the advice in this book comes in. Followed correctly, there is no doubt that it will help you.

The first part of the book, written primarily by myself, Ken Hambly, is an explanation not just of autonomic overload, but the way you look at events, and how these perceptions affect your body. It's about the interface between your environment at home or at work, and your body's mechanisms for interpreting this external world and responding to it.

The second half, written mainly by Alice Muir, is designed to help you learn to manage your autonomic overload. It is intended to empower you to improve the quality of your life and the quality of the lives of those who care about you and are close to you – not just now, but permanently.

If you follow the principles set out in this book carefully and honestly, they will help you fulfil your potential so that your own abilities, your natural confidence and true competence will shine through. If you think that you appear to others to be less than you really are, then now's the time to do something about it.

The steps you will take to achieve a relaxed, comfortable, high-performing life are practical and straightforward, but take effort, as it does to break any bad habit, such as smoking. You have to work at it systematically and diligently with no backsliding or short cuts. There is no gain without pain, and there is nothing passive in this protocol.

Dealing with your problem by yourself is perfectly possible, but it is much easier to get it under control if you have someone to help you. That may be a partner who has read and understood this book, or it might be a professional person trained to give you advice and help with this type of problem and who has suitable qualifications. It takes time, and such people are hard to find in the NHS or conventional medical situations.

Above all, do not, definitely do not, go through your life underachieving. Even if you do seem to achieve a lot at work or in other ways, it may be at great personal cost, and you may still be underachieving. Perhaps you really should be the company chairman. Why should a less able person do that job when it should be you? Perhaps you feel anxious in a supermarket and uncomfortable in crowded places. Don't accept that – don't put up with it. Do something about it, and do it now. We understand how you feel and why you feel the way you do, and we do have answers to your problems.

2

Autonomic Overload – How It Works

You don't need a medical degree to understand your autonomic nervous system, but you do need an open mind and curiosity about the way your body works. The direct cause of these symptoms and difficulties lies within your body, and in particular in your nervous system and the way it reacts to the outside world. However, your nervous system perceives and interprets the outside world through your brain.

What is autonomic overload?

Your autonomic nervous system is by far the largest and most important part of your whole nervous system. The word 'autonomic' in Greek means 'self-governing', and refers to the nervous control of your body which works all by itself without any help from you – in fact you should be completely unaware of the actions of your autonomic nervous system, which performs miracles of command and control every second of our lives. Do you have to tell your body to breathe in and breathe out? Do you have to decide on an appropriate heart rate? Do you have to decide to sweat if you are in a hot environment or if you are exercising? Certainly not. Your autonomic nervous system looks after you very well and performs all of these tasks for you, all by itself. We can focus our eyes, stand up or sit down, breathe and our heart can beat all because of the unconscious actions of this important part of the body's systems which is pre-programmed to adjust itself according to circumstances as well as co-ordinating the routine tasks to keep you alive. All this goes on without us knowing anything about it – until of course it goes wrong.

Adapting

Most of the time our bodies respond very quickly to external events which we see or hear, such as a loud noise which makes us 'jump'. The automatic response of your nervous system means adapting your internal environment according to external forces – for example, if you walk up a steep slope, by increasing your breathing rate and heart rate. It's like having all your thermostats set right and adjusted correctly to keep everything working normally.

Much of this adaptation happens automatically, using sensors that detect changes in your temperature or measure the oxygen saturation of your blood, and alter your metabolism and breathing rate to correct these changes. In this way your body is 'self governing', using your autonomic nervous system to control this internal environment. It isn't all completely automatic, however. Sometimes your body has to interpret the external environment using your eyes and ears and touch, and these perceptions are moderated and transmitted through another important part of your nervous system – your brain. Your brain isn't automatic: it thinks. Sometimes it thinks too much.

Where is the autonomic nervous system?

That isn't easy to demonstrate. It is a system rather than one organ, and it occurs throughout the body. It is a mixture of nerves, connections and glands. It involves areas of the brain, much of the spinal cord and nerve connections elsewhere, and also glands that pump hormones into the blood stream. It is an integral part of the body and it works in conjunction with just about every other system that we have.

Basically, problems often start when the part of the brain that controls the 'fight-or-flight' mechanism starts firing at an abnormally high rate, releasing neurotransmitters such as norepinephrine – chemicals usually released by the nervous system in response to short-term stress. When the stress continues too long, this chemical message can swamp the system, leading to autonomic overload and making the brain more sensitive to firing off again in response to a stimulus, even if you are not in imminent danger.

Problems

One of the main functions of the autonomic nervous system is to deal instantly with perceived threats. When there is danger, all sorts of 'booster' systems come into play which physically tone up your body and make it respond. It is an amazing and complex system essential to our survival both as individuals and as a species, but it can cause problems.

The entire system usually works very well, unbelievably so, responding to real and imminent physical danger. But what is danger? At which level of danger will these booster systems kick in? How do we perceive danger and how do we interpret the signs and sounds of danger in our environment? We have to make judgements about that and judgements are made in our brain at a conscious level, so that for some people even the thought of danger will trigger an autonomic response. Their heart may speed up and they may sweat, for example. When we ourselves, via our brain, intervene and start to mitigate and interpret the environment in which we live, we are in a whole new ball game. Our autonomic nervous system now responds to what we think, rather than to what it detects through its sensors.

Many of you will know how it works. Some dogs, for example, sleep through fireworks and thunder or people shouting while others are nervy, jumpy and instantly run away from loud noises, which tells us one of two things. Either they have a very responsive automatic nervous system, or else they see danger in everything, perhaps having an inappropriate idea of what danger is. In either case, their body reacts to facilitate a physical response in different situations and one dog responds more quickly and more actively in a situation than another. People are like dogs.

These responses can be learned through past experiences, but also, dogs are born with different tolerances to perceived threats. In the evolutionary process the dog with the more active autonomic nervous system may be more successful at surviving because it can respond more quickly than its colleague who remains asleep. The 'nervous' dog has a more efficient flight-or-fight reaction. Its body is ready quicker than another dog for whatever is to come.

The human response

Enough about dogs! We brainy and intellectual humans respond in exactly the same way, but perhaps with worse potential complications because we think more. We learn more complex things, and we imagine more complex situations than simple animals. We intellectualize danger and see threats where there may be none, and we have to deal with problems like public speaking, or coping with debt, or with an unfaithful partner, which feel like danger to us because they threaten our lifestyle, if not our actual lives.

Our thought processes are more complex, but our autonomic nervous system is essentially the same. We have this brain full of problems, real or sometimes imagined or exaggerated, charging up the network of nerves and glands that we call our autonomic nervous system. Should we be surprised if occasionally it becomes overloaded in either the short or the long term?

The steady state

Now you have that image – our brain buzzing with problems and an autonomic nervous system, that self-governing controller of all our body, trying to hold it all together in a steady state. Our body chemistry, temperature, the working of our intestines or bladder and all the rest, must be kept right. When there are too many strong messages from the brain to the autonomic nervous system, when it is pushed too far, then autonomic overload occurs.

We are all susceptible to this problem, some more than others by virtue of inherited characteristics or childhood impressions, or both, but everyone has a point at which autonomic overload kicks in and things start to go wrong. Our nervous system gets its wires crossed, transmits the wrong instructions and we start to get symptoms – physical, psychological or behavioural (see Chapters 3, 4 and 5). These symptoms can thus make us perform less well, and worry more about our decreasing performance. Our body is no longer in a steady state, it is in free fall. You may well know what that feels like.

Now what?

You will be pleased to know that you have already begun your treatment. In fact you are a long way down the treatment road. You decided to buy or read this book about your problems and if you have read this far you have learned quite a lot about why you get symptoms. You will know that you are not alone.

Step one of almost any treatment is understanding, and you will already have an understanding of the sort of mechanisms which produce your problems. With this knowledge, you will be able to understand and assimilate other facts about the way your body works.

Understanding, though, is not enough – it can be hugely disappointing to understand the nature of your problem and then find that you can't make it go away. You have to have a system for tackling the problem, and that is what we aim to provide in this book. So now please read on!

3

How Do You Feel Today?

When you suffer from autonomic overload you usually do not feel well; in fact, you may feel ill most of the time and that isn't pleasant. Feeling unwell is a problem in itself, but it's made worse if you don't know why, and no one can explain why you feel the way you do. Other emotions and worries take over and add to your problems, so that you begin to feel progressively worse.

You want to do the things you have always been able to do, but you know that it will be difficult, so you settle for less. That is one of the principal consequences of this condition, you accept a less satisfactory lifestyle than you should, and you are less fulfilled and you enjoy life less. Of course you can cope, you can manage, but it's always an effort. The pleasure factor is removed from many activities. You may go to a party or a social event, but you do so with clenched teeth and every action is an effort. Eventually you may begin to feel that it just isn't worthwhile making the effort and begin to live a life which is less satisfactory than it should be.

Your day

It's hard to explain the way you feel to other people, even those close to you who may love you and care about you. Autonomic overload is a very private thing, in the sense that it is hard to communicate to others what it is actually like on a day-to-day basis.

So you get up in the morning stiff and sore, and you struggle through your day. Your symptoms are intrusive and unpleasant, but usually manageable. So you manage without complaint. If things are going well you may not be so bad, and cope reasonably well. If you are stressed then your symptoms are much worse. We all find some situations difficult, and some more difficult to deal with than others, and the prospect of having to deal with these problems makes life intolerable. Some days are full of situations like this, and on these days life just makes us feel ill.

Tiredness is cumulative. Stressful events can make us feel worse and increase our autonomic overload; physical stress such as cold weather outside or a cold room, or the physical effects of our overload such as colicky pain or an upset stomach can increase our psychological pain. You can always cope, but some days are simply worse than others.

It isn't usually the events of a bad day which cause the problems – very often, it's the anticipation of these events. On a day with a challenging event, we may wake up feeling terrible even before we remember the meeting or the speech or whatever it is which may be the cause of our problem. Our body is there before us. Our autonomic overload is up and running before we are aware of the reason.

Life events

No, not major life events. Not death or divorce, but day-to-day events can seem too much, and we may fear we won't be able to manage. We fear that the tiredness will overwhelm us. Our irritable bowel syndrome becomes intolerable. We get leg or chest pain. We may start to feel panicky in some places. It is the extreme reactivity of our sensitized autonomic nervous system which has taken over our lives.

Once our autonomic nervous system overreacts, simple life events like a visit to the cinema become a nightmare.

Going out

Let's look at that visit to the cinema. What are the dynamics of that situation? Well, for you it may be no trouble at all. One person's nightmare can be another person's enjoyable night out. Let's assume that you do have problems in public places. It isn't unusual and for people with autonomic overload it is very common. If you have agreed to go to the cinema in the evening you can wake up feeling ill. You don't know why, you just do. Your autonomic nervous system is firing on all cylinders and you don't even know why. Then you remember – you are going out that evening. It might be the cinema, the theatre, a party or just a night with friends. Whatever it is, it has triggered part of that dreaded 'fight-or-flight' reaction. Your autonomic nervous system is up and running.

Why do you feel bad? Check it out. You are tight. Your jaw

muscles, shoulder muscles, all your muscles are sore and tense. You might feel sick due to having too much acid in your stomach. You will have a tremor due to muscle tension. As the day wears on other symptoms develop, slightly different for everyone. Needless to say, you begin to feel apprehensive, even frightened. The old 'what if?' thought starts to intrude into your life. What if something happens (and you can choose anything you like so long as it is likely to embarrass you and make you conspicuous)? Psychological and physical symptoms combine to make you very uncomfortable.

By the time you are supposed to be going out it seems that you will simply be unable to do it. You may have diarrhoea or be passing water all the time, just due to an overactive bowel and a tense bladder. Your imagination goes wild and you imagine all sorts of possible disasters. People round about you may become irritable, often genuinely unable to understand what is happening. Perhaps surprisingly, you always do manage to go out as planned, despite your fears. It's almost as if you know that even though you have a physical awareness and experience of your fear, you also know that it is a paper tiger and will not actually do you any harm.

The desire to conform is paramount in a herd animal such as we are, so we do conform and we do go out as planned. We also know that it will be all right, that we will cope and more than that, we may even be the life and soul of the party. If we get to the cinema, the first quarter of an hour will be bad. The second quarter of an hour will be a little better, and the rest of the evening will be fine. It always works that way. You can go out, and you can enjoy the experience. It is often the anticipation and the early adjustment to the loud, strange and intimidating environment that causes the trouble.

A different day?

In the end, your day wasn't too bad. You forced yourself to go out and it may even have been quite enjoyable. But wouldn't it be nice if you could have a different day? A day that wasn't, frankly, ruined by nervous anticipation and unpleasant physical symptoms? A day when you felt relaxed, healthy, fulfilled and free to be yourself, without any dread or hard work at all? It is possible.

Our message is, be all that you can be. Don't settle for second best. You may feel that you have a severe problem which other people don't seem to experience and don't understand. However, many people do suffer the way you do, and manage to overcome it. You can do the same – so why not accept the challenge and strive for a better life. Keep at it for as long as it takes. Make it an important part of your life, because the potential rewards are great indeed. Perhaps at the moment you simply do not know what is at the end of the rainbow, and may have no idea what your life could be like. You do not know what you could make it be like. It's time you found out. The secret is quiet perseverance – so now please read on. The next two chapters are going to look in more detail at symptoms you might experience, and will help you collect the evidence you need to start changing your life – and your day.

4

Psychological Symptoms

Psychological symptoms are one of the main problems of autonomic overload. They may only last a while in the form of fleeting panic, or they may have been present for as long as you can remember and feel like ingrained anxiety. You may have seen a doctor about them; you may even have had them investigated in hospital in case there was a physical problem such as thyroid disease, but there is every chance that no cause was found. Even worse, it is unlikely that any explanation was offered. You may have some idea about what is going on yourself, but it is very unlikely that anyone has made any suggestions about what you can do about it.

It is important to appreciate that psychological symptoms may vary in type and severity. They may be severe and almost disabling, or they may be low key and chronic, just enough to interfere with your life to a significant degree and make you behave in a way which doesn't do you justice. These symptoms may be related to certain threatening situations, often social situations or at work, so that you avoid doing the very things you would like to do and know that you could do. These effects are not bizarre, random and unrelated, as you may think, but logical and understandable and you should never feel embarrassed about having them. They simply indicate that you have a sensitive, functioning autonomic nervous system – as have many people from the beginning of time, often to their advantage in a more primitive world!

You may recognize some of the symptoms in this chapter – but don't panic, no one with autonomic overload will ever suffer from all of them at once, and they vary in severity, or change from time to time. All are normal reactions which everyone experiences from time to time, though they may be a bit more severe in some situations than most people experience. So relax a bit about your symptoms. Okay, you may be mentally uncomfortable or, worse, feeling worried and upset, but *there is nothing fundamentally wrong with you.* That is our basic message. This book will give you a logical way to manage this overactive nervous system.

Anxiety and anticipation

These are probably the two most common psychological problems of autonomic overload. Your anxiety can be acute and short-lived, and everyone experiences that in extreme situations so it is normal, but what if you are anxious all the time, or anxious at minor social events? What if your anxiety is just ordinary anxiety, but it occurs in an extraordinary way? Your anxiety may be out of control, and it may come to dominate your life.

We all know about feeling anxious before an event such as public speaking, and having feelings of tummy upset, or a hand tremor. There is a close association between psychological problems and perceptions and physical reactions. Strangely, they are often worse before an event and get better during the event.

Anticipation is just anxiety misbehaving. Your anxiety about a coming event may begin days or weeks in advance and start to affect many aspects of your life. You may feel anxious and not know why. You may be born an anxious person, perhaps as a result of childhood experiences, perhaps as a result of a low threshold for anxiety. If it is related to particular situations you could call this a phobia.

Depression

Everyone can feel a little 'down', particularly if they don't feel physically well or if circumstances are difficult. There is a fundamental difference between this transient feeling and the kind of depression which is overwhelming and destructive – when you feel that you are in a hole and can't get out, or see the future. You might feel that life isn't worth living and even have thoughts of harming yourself. This is a potentially serious problem for which you should seek help from your doctor. It is important that you do this for two reasons. The first is that it might get worse and cause you real problems later, and the second is that depression is treatable with medication.

Do not ignore depression, or underestimate it. The advice and exercises in this book may help you and you can certainly use them, but only after you have consulted a doctor and considered other options.

Panic disorder

For some people the feeling of panic, or impending panic, is predominant. You may feel panicky most of the time, but it is worse in confined places, public transport or in supermarkets. You may have a panic attack (or attacks) where you are suddenly overwhelmed by a feeling of pure panic. You get a rapid heart rate, feel sweaty and faint. This is pure autonomic overload and demonstrates the association between perceived danger, a mental exercise, and a physical response. It's like flicking a switch. It feels like the end of the world, but in fact it only lasts a few seconds before it fades away leaving you uncomfortable, exhausted and fearful. While you may have an inbuilt tendency to be like this, at times of stress your autonomic nervous system is overloaded and you will be more panicky more often.

In reality nothing very much has happened to you and you will never come to any harm from a panic attack. You won't faint or shout out or do anything silly. If you don't choose to show that you are having a panic attack then you could carry on a conversation with someone and they would never know. It feels terrible of course, it is really testing and there is a strong impulse to run out of the shop, theatre or wherever, but you probably won't do that and you probably never will. The need to conform is much too strong for that and it overcomes the need to react to panic. People feel panicky in aircraft, but they don't try to get off! They don't make fools of themselves. People conform no matter how bad they feel. In Chapter 11 we will give you advice about how to manage panic attacks.

Phobias

Well, everyone knows what a phobia is – don't they? A phobia is an irrational fear of something, isn't it? Well no, it isn't, actually. A person who has a phobia is someone who gets powerful, disturbing and possibly disabling symptoms in particular situations to which they are sensitized, just as if they were allergic to them. As these symptoms are often very powerful, what could be more sensible or logical? As in a panic attack, the symptoms are real, not imagined, and powerful, not exaggerated. There is nothing irrational about a phobia – anyone experiencing these powerful symptoms would be

23

distressed by them, and the phobia is often fairly logical in developmental terms. What could be more logical than getting a surge of autonomic activity when confronted by a snake? Any animal would react in that way, and the stronger the autonomic response the better that animal's chance of survival. Flight or fight!

We are animals, of course. We are mammals and we respond like other mammals. We are programmed to respond in particular ways, so that our reaction is automatic, rapid and potentially life-saving. That is what the autonomic nervous system is for, to give us an instantaneous reaction, unplanned by us and self-governing, even though in a phobia it appears to occur to excess.

The human factor

The factor which makes us slightly different from other mammals is the way our brain works. We think, we imagine, we live in a sophisticated social environment with financial, work and domestic pressures which pump up our autonomic nervous system to a degree which makes it perform inappropriately. It becomes too 'trigger happy' and fires off too easily in these circumstances. We can be phobic about ideas and thoughts, just as we can feel panicky about ideas and thoughts. These mental concepts are transmitted to our autonomic nervous system by several very clever methods producing an instantaneous physical response. This is exactly what is intended – remember that flight-or-fight reaction? It is about survival. It's about living to fight another day, or at least about living.

We see danger in places other animals don't. We see danger at work or at social events or in aircraft or shops. But is that correct? Most animals would see danger in a plane or in a supermarket, or often in a thunderstorm. In fact we are just like our fellow creatures and our autonomic response is quite normal in one sense. We have actually failed to suppress logical symptoms intended to save our life, which rather turns the concept of a phobia on its head. Perhaps the person with the phobia is right, and everyone else is wrong. Perhaps a phobia is a proper use of our autonomic nervous system, and it is the rest of us who will be bitten by snakes and spiders or trapped in lifts or planes. Never, ever feel embarrassed or guilty about the things you feel or the way your body behaves. Look on a phobia as a survival instinct gone haywire.

Obsessive-compulsive disorders (OCD)

OCD can take a number of forms, but is basically the feeling that you need to keep doing the same thing over and over again, often hand-washing or other acts related to cleanliness. Sometimes it is the repetition of unwanted thoughts or ideas that seem to occur over and over again, like a tune that goes round and round in your head.

Many of us have these feelings from time to time and it is rarely a problem, but if you think that it's a problem for you or that it is getting worse, seek medical advice. The advice in this book isn't enough to properly manage this type of difficulty. Such psychological disorders can be made worse by strain on your autonomic nervous system, but they fall into a specialist category and are not really part of our story.

Loss of confidence

This is hardly a symptom, it is a fact of life. If you have so many apparently different problems going on, you probably won't feel as confident as you would like. Autonomic overload can affect our performance and efficiency, and that doesn't help our confidence. So a lack of confidence can be the result of the way your body reacts, or of the way you think about yourself, or your ability to concentrate and perform tasks. If you get some of your symptoms in particular situations you will certainly not be confident or comfortable in these situations, and you may even begin to avoid them. Once you start to lose confidence it can last a lifetime, but confidence is recoverable.

What is confidence? Surely confidence is a lack of autonomic symptoms in all situations. If you get nausea, a tremor, feel shaky or have a headache you won't be as confident as someone who doesn't have these physical problems. You may even begin to feel inadequate compared to other people. That doesn't mean that you are less able or less competent than they are and you may well overcompensate and actually perform very well, but at a cost to yourself. You may have to work harder at it than a very confident person, but then there are compensations for being the way you are. Overconfident people tend to be pushy and may not be generally liked. If you are under-confident you may have empathy and understanding, and a generous spirit appreciated by others.

No doubt you would like to be more confident, and the way to achieve that is to deal with the various problems you may have which together add up to a lack of confidence. This book will help you to do this by dealing with the way you think and the way you see yourself and others.

What can I do?

Check yourself out. You may have had psychological symptoms for so long that you have become used to them. You put up with them, disregard them and may have become unaware of what is happening. Take a critical look at the way you feel in all situations, every aspect of your life as you are going about your business. Ask yourself: 'How do I feel mentally?' Are you comfortable with yourself or are you ill at ease? Are you depressed? Are you irritable and snappy with the people around you? Do you have problems relating to others, or difficulties with relationships at work?

All of these are important areas of your life, and they should be working for you as well as they can do. You can't of course change your basic personality. You were born to be the way that you are, but you should be comfortable with that person and fulfil your potential both emotionally and in the real world. Autonomic problems are not an essential part of your persona. You may have been born with a tendency to be susceptible to anxiety or stress, but you can deal with that if you go about it the right way, and this book will show you the way. You can shed these hindrances to the fulfilment of your potential and really be yourself. That is what is on offer.

What if?

One of the recurring thoughts which gives most trouble is the dreaded 'What if?' rumination. Some of us constantly ask: 'What if something happens?' 'What if I shout out?' 'What if I forget what I was going to say during my presentation?'

There are a million 'What ifs?' in every situation, and everyone has these thoughts. Some of us have them more than others, and if they become intrusive you may have a problem. Later we will see what we can do about that. For now, have a look at the way you think. Do you ask yourself the 'What if?' question? Do you have a rational view of your own ability? Do you talk yourself down so that you will not be able to fulfil your potential?

Thinking problems

Perhaps you are constantly thinking that other people can do something, but you really can't. You may have unreal ideas about the nature of your ability and what you should be able to do. You may constantly feel let down, thinking that you 'Ought to be able to do that' or that you 'Should be able to do something!'

Why make these assumptions about what other people can do and what you ought or should be able to do? Who says that you have to do anything, or that you should be able to do something? Are these ideas rational? You might be living in a world of false expectations or unrealistic ideas. You may have problems with the way you think about things. You aren't mad. You don't think that you are Napoleon, but you may not have realistic expectations about your life and potential either. You may underestimate yourself, or you might overestimate yourself.

Know yourself

It is important to know about yourself. The more you can learn about the way you feel and think and the way your body responds the easier it will be to get a handle on your problems and begin to sort them out. Make a note on paper, or just start to pay conscious attention to the way you feel and the person you are. It's a simple thing you can start now, so why not do it? Just raise your awareness a little, just become conscious of the things that are going on in your everyday life. It will affect your curiosity and it will be of interest because you have never looked at these things before. What you find might surprise you.

5

Physical Symptoms

The autonomic nervous system is where the body and brain, the internal and external environment come together. It is the 'nerve centre' of the organism which is you, the place that makes things happen. Yet strangely it isn't exactly a place, it isn't a black box where connections are made as in a car, or even in a computer. Nor is it simply a wiring loom; it is a combination of nervous and glandular systems throughout your body which work all by themselves to keep your body functioning at its very best. Your autonomic nervous system keeps you in a steady state, and if there is a need due to danger, it gives that steady state a shove so that it works at a higher level of physical response.

The need can be a sudden exposure to danger requiring a physical response, or it may be some kind of slow background emotional or physical stress. This stress will push your autonomic nervous system and make it overreact and overstimulate your body systems, and thus instead of producing a beneficial short-term physical effect, autonomic overload in the longer term produces physical symptoms which can be severe and distressing, and in the very long term dangerous.

This chapter looks at some of the physical symptoms often associated with an overactive autonomic nervous system. Remember that this list isn't exhaustive and that there might be other causes for some of the symptoms listed. Remember also that these are functional symptoms, disorders of your normal bodily function, which in that sense are not abnormal at all, just variations on the normal. No one, no matter how confident and contained, is immune to at least a brief episode of autonomic overload, so these symptoms can occur briefly to anyone.

Problems with muscles or joints

The main physical problem with an overloaded autonomic nervous system tends to be pain, with muscle tension and physical exhaustion often being the main causes.

Pain is due to excess tension in muscles, including the muscles of the neck producing tension headaches. Excessive muscle tension leads to excessive fatigue. The muscular pain is worst and typically occurs in the neck and shoulders, but it can be felt anywhere – the arms or legs or in the back. Pain and stiffness are almost routine in autonomic overload.

The pain is caused by tension or tightness in muscles which goes on for 24 hours a day, even when you are asleep. You can wake up in the morning with a sore neck and shoulders, a sore jaw from teeth clenching through the night, and nail marks on the palms of your hands from fist clenching. Have you been sleeping in a relaxed way? Are you refreshed and ready for the new day? Perhaps not!

Tetany

Tetany is a condition of extreme muscle spasm often experienced by young people, particularly young girls who hyperventilate. Most people will know that when this happens the 'first aid' of choice is to breathe into a paper bag. Tetany is thought of as an acute problem of short duration, usually hysterical in nature. The physiological mechanism involved will be discussed later, but for now it is enough to know that it isn't uncommon and that it is usually an isolated occurrence.

Tetany can be chronic, that is to say it can be low level, long-lasting and constant. It is tetany which produces much of the muscle pain that people with autonomic overload experience. It is due to chronic hyperventilation, a less well understood part of autonomic overload. So tetany has a very important role in the generation of physical symptoms.

Headache

Tension headaches are caused by tightness in the muscles of your neck. You may be able to feel the tension if you press on the tight muscles in the front and back of your neck with your thumbs – indeed, the pain can be excruciating. If you feel across your neck you may be able to identify little knots in the muscles at the back, and if you press on these you may experience extreme pain. You may also feel a little dizzy as if you might be going to fall to the side, but the mechanism again is muscle tension.

Many people think they are having a migraine because the pain is so severe, but migraines are quite different in character, often being one-sided and associated with vomiting. Tension headaches really can last for days and be almost disabling during that time.

Back and leg pain

We have muscles everywhere, in our chest and in our legs, arms and back. When we are in a state of autonomic overload all muscles are susceptible to tension, tenderness and pain, so we may get back pain or leg pain or cramps. The pain fits the pattern, it is all caused by the same phenomenon. It is caused by the hyperventilation, or over-breathing (see tetany above). The pain does not respond well to painkillers, particularly those with codeine, but it does respond to the general treatment of autonomic overload we outline in this book. Remember that the key to the treatment of all conditions is the same, so it isn't a matter of treating each individual problem; it's the treatment of the whole person and the whole problem that is the answer. That makes the whole thing so much easier.

Neurological problems

Neurological problems are problems to do with the brain and the nervous system. Or rather, they seem to be to do with the brain and the nervous system, but as always they are simply due to overactivity of the nervous system due to autonomic overload. They may also have a psychological element such as worry, and it may be the worry which triggers the autonomic response.

Strange feelings

Sometimes people feel a little unreal or detached. They may just feel a little odd, and then there are the psychological problems such as anxiety and uncertainty which can just make someone feel unsteady or uncomfortable. This is not necessarily just a physical problem, it is part of the complex emotional and psychological reaction to your autonomic overload and none of these symptoms can do you any harm, so for now just live with them. Again, these feelings will respond to the general treatment of your autonomic overload.

Faintness

Sometimes people feel faint. This may be because they get palpitations or suddenly feel a little queasy, or perhaps they just feel a little panicky. There can be all sorts of reasons but someone with autonomic overload won't faint. Technically a faint occurs when there is a fall in blood pressure and a resulting decrease in the blood flow to the brain. When that happens there is an actual loss of consciousness and the person will fall down. It happens in warm places or at times when the circulation has opened up for some reason such as pregnancy.

There is no such mechanism operating in the case of someone with autonomic overload, so while such a person may faint for the usual reasons just like anyone else, your autonomic overload per se will never make you faint.

Dizziness and unsteadiness

As with fainting there can be many reasons for a feeling of unsteadiness, but that's all it is, a feeling. You won't reel about or fall over. If you do, there is something else causing the problem and you should seek medical help. The sensation is very different from that of vertigo where there is a rotational effect and you will fall down if you don't hold on to something. If you have experienced both you will know what the difference is.

The usual reason for this feeling of unsteadiness is spasm in the muscles on one side of your neck which is greater than the tension in the muscles on the other side. Your neck muscles are involved in your sense of position, of where your head is, and so if this is upset you feel as if you are going to one side. In fact you aren't, and you can walk in a straight line. If you feel dizzy in this way, do a little test. Press the muscles in your neck with your thumb as before and see if you are more tense on one side than the other. See if pressing on these tense muscles makes you feel more dizzy. Like so many of the frightening symptoms you can get, there is a perfectly logical and simple explanation. The degree of distress you feel is considerable, but the actual cause is really a minor dysfunction of one of your body's systems. Again, it is an exaggeration of something which is normal.

Difficulty with concentration and memory

Well, with all this going on in your internal environment how could you be expected to concentrate? We are talking about overload, and your brain is overloaded with worries and problems, immediate worries about what might happen in the next few minutes. You become absorbed in your internal environment – the working of your body – so that you are aware of every physical thing that is happening. You concentrate on this, not on someone's small talk or what you had for breakfast. No wonder you have problems with concentration and memory. It is entirely understandable and normal. It may be something you have to put up with until it settles down.

Respiratory (Breathing)

Cough. People with autonomic overload may get a cough or 'tickle' in their throat. The tickle makes them cough; the more they cough the worse the tickle becomes, and so on until the cough itself is a bit of a problem. Solve the problems with the nervous overload and this will, like all the rest of these problems, simply disappear. Other reasons for a cough include medication and, if it is moist and productive, chest problems. A cough which is unexplained can be functional and may even become a habit.

Shortness of breath. This problem is known to doctors as 'atypical asthma' though it has nothing to do with real asthma where the breathing tubes close down. With atypical asthma there is no actual cause for the problem, but you are aware of a sensation of being short of breath. There are some people who get up at night and throw open the windows to allow more air into the room, though there is certainly enough air already in the room for a football team to breathe. Read the next section.

Tightness in the chest. Isn't it strange how often muscle tightness plays a major part in the problems of people with autonomic overload? Here is another one: you just feel that you can't get a full breath. No matter how hard you try, you can never completely fill your lungs. You chest feels tight, but if a doctor was to listen to your chest with a stethoscope there would be nothing abnormal to hear and a chest X-ray would be normal. You would have 'normal air entry' and the doctor would be perplexed.

How could you explain this strange and disturbing sensation? With the knowledge you have already gained you might well be able to work it out. The problem lies in the increased muscle tension you have in the muscles of your chest wall, those muscles between your ribs and in your back. It is tightness in muscles again causing problems. It is the muscles in your chest wall between your ribs and not the muscles of your bronchioles (your breathing tubes) which are in spasm, so as you try to take a deep breath, you feel constricted, you just can't get a full breath. You feel as if there is a tight band round your chest, stopping you from breathing. Again it is a simple and understandable problem entirely in keeping with your underlying autonomic overload. It isn't permanent, it isn't dangerous, it's uncomfortable and possibly a little frightening but nothing more.

Sighing – excessive yawning. This is common in people suffering from autonomic overload, and it has an important part to play in the generation of many of the symptoms we have mentioned. Everyone who has these autonomic problems breathes more deeply than 'normal', and many will sigh more and some will yawn a lot. The need to breathe more rapidly or more deeply is rooted in the fight-or-flight reaction where a good supply of oxygen in the blood is necessary if you are to do either. If you are pressured or stressed, you will tend to overbreathe and sigh or yawn.

This sighing, yawning and any overbreathing are thus a direct result of pressure on your autonomic nervous system, and as it is important it will be discussed at length later. However, paradoxically, though this problem is important in the production of symptoms, you probably aren't aware that you are doing it.

To find out if you do sigh a lot, put a hand on your chest while you are watching TV and feel the rise and fall of your chest wall. You may notice that you sigh a lot or take a lot of deep breaths.

Heart and circulation

About 50 per cent of medical patients referred to a hospital cardiologist, or heart specialist, don't have cardiac problems at all. They have cardiac 'symptoms', but no cause is found after extensive investigation. How can this be? If these patients have functional symptoms, what treatment is offered? The answer often is – none at all. You're on your own.

The autonomic nervous system has a direct effect on the heart and circulation, as we will find out later. Adrenaline, a neurotransmitter in the autonomic nervous system, works directly on the heart, mainly to make it speed up in an emergency. If your autonomic nervous system is in overload then adrenaline and other mechanisms such as direct nervous control will obviously have an effect on the heart, making it go too fast or skip beats, which can be very disturbing.

If you have problems which seem to be related to your heart you should of course see your doctor. An electrocardiogram is a simple test which can usually sort out any problems and may be reassuring. If it is normal and your doctor is satisfied that there is nothing serious to worry about, you might consider the following:

Fast heart rate. Some people may notice that their heart is racing, going so fast that they become aware of its beat. This may happen in some difficult situations or it may come out of the blue. As with so many other symptoms this does not mean that there is anything wrong with the heart, it's simply that the heart is going faster than usual. Anyone's heart rate can vary, so this is simply a deviation from the norm. If, of course it became extreme, and you would be aware of the difference, then there might be a physical cause and you might need medical help. If it is a simple speeding up of the heart then it will settle down by itself if you relax.

Palpitations. When you get palpitations, and just about everyone does at some time in their lives, your heart becomes irregular. It tends to put in a few extra beats and then it misses a beat so that there is a gap and you are left with a funny feeling in your chest for a second. It can be quite disturbing and quite prolonged, but it is due to the effect of adrenaline on the heart and not to any problem with the heart itself. If it becomes a regular occurrence then you might need to see a doctor and possibly have a cardiogram, but palpitations by themselves can do you no harm.

Chest pain. Chest pain should be taken seriously and if severe you should seek immediate medical assistance, possibly via an emergency ambulance. If you do have chest pain and it has been thoroughly assessed and investigated by a doctor and nothing wrong is found, and you still have the pain, then it may be due to other causes unrelated to your heart. It could be due to the muscles in your chest wall, again being overly tense, or it could be due to too much acid in your stomach. It might be due to pain in the small joints of your chest wall where your ribs join your breastbone. These things may be made worse by autonomic overload with its associated over-breathing.

Stomach and intestines

Everyone knows that in difficult situations you can get diarrhoea, or feel sick. Anyone who has had to make a speech knows how upset their stomach can get. These things are normal in difficult situations but for some people they can become a habit. In the immediate situation when danger threatens, your body does everything it can to help you with the fight-or-flight reaction, and that includes dumping anything the body does not need. You will experience a physical reaction intended to empty the bowel of its contents and also the bladder. In a dangerous situation that would be normal, but with long-term chronic overload it leads to unwanted, often familiar symptoms.

Oral dryness. Or dry mouth. When you are nervous you tend to get a dry mouth. Your tongue sticks to the roof of your mouth, you have no saliva, and you feel as if you won't be able to talk. This is a common problem, though usually very short-lived.

Stomach pain. By this we mean pain in your anatomical stomach, under your ribs and in the middle, sometimes going up into your chest. It is due to having too much acid in your stomach. And why do you get too much acid? It's all due to autonomic overload: here, the 'motor' nerve (in this case the vagus nerve), which causes glands in the stomach to secrete strong hydrochloric acid, forces the glands to produce more acid than usual. It burns your stomach and gullet and you get pain. It can be of short duration, or it can last a long time. In the latter case you need to have a medical opinion about it.

Intestinal cramps. Here we are bordering on the problem of the Irritable Bowel Syndrome, a condition not uncommon in autonomic overload. Your intestine depends upon a wave of contraction starting at the top and sweeping right through to the other end, thus carrying the intestinal contents through the gut. If this does not happen in a co-ordinated way, when one part of the intestine contracts against another, then there can be severe crampy pain. Ask any baby! Babies have an immature nervous system so that their bowel tends to lack co-ordination and they get colic. In this situation where co-ordination is compromised due to an overactive autonomic nervous system, there can be diarrhoea or constipation with crampy pain and bloating – your tummy becomes distended.

Altered bowel habit. This means diarrhoea or constipation as discussed above. In all of these situations you have to exercise some common sense. If you have severe bowel symptoms or if there is associated weight loss or any other symptoms then you obviously must see a doctor and have some simple investigations performed. If your symptoms are short lived, or if your investigations are negative, then the cause may be autonomic overload. If this is the case then the approach outlined in this book may help you.

Swallowing problems

Some people experience problems swallowing. They feel that there is a ball in their gullet and they just can't swallow it no matter how hard they try. The technical name is *globus hystericus* and it is as old as medicine itself – or perhaps as old as humankind itself. Forget about the word 'hystericus', that has historical relevance. This tight ball in your gullet is – well, you should have guessed it – it's muscle spasm due to autonomic overload. It's similar to tightness in the chest or to intestinal cramps. It happens when you are under pressure, at a meeting or a party, and it is very unpleasant. There is of course nothing physical, or pathological, wrong with you. It is a functional disorder. It is tension in muscles. It will go away.

In the immediate situation the more you try to swallow the worse it will become. The answer is to try to relax and breathe slowly and let the swallowing take care of itself. More about this approach later.

Bladder problems

Isn't it interesting how many of these problems occur in what doctors call a 'hollow viscus', meaning a tube or a vessel? The intestine is a tube, the gullet is a tube and the stomach and bladder are really vessels. They are all lined by muscles which can expand or contract, and which should do that in a co-ordinated and organized way. If you want to pass water, you relax the muscles of the bladder neck which keep the urine in – and contract the muscles of the bladder wall which squeeze it out. Think about it. That is how we empty our bladders. How is it co-ordinated? By your autonomic nervous system of course – that is its function, that's what it is for. Your thinking brain can't think of all these things in sequence and instruct the muscles to do the job. Think of what you would have to do just to stand up. It all happens magically, through the unconscious functioning or your self-governing nervous system.

Your bladder is just the same. When things are going well it functions perfectly and you know nothing about it. When things are going wrong, then you can have all sorts of problems. The muscles may be too tight, or they may contract in the wrong sequence, and you can become uncomfortable.

Frequency. This is the most common problem and it means passing water too often. You may want to go all the time, or you may feel the need to go when you go out or to a public event. To make matters worse, autonomic problems may increase the amount of urine you produce in your kidneys so that you do have to go more often, but this is not the main reason for your distress. It is usually that old problem of muscle spasm making you feel as if you want to go more often.

Men in particular can experience an unpleasant feeling after passing water. A few drops of urine can become trapped in the tube to the outside and cause intense irritation as your muscles contract. This problem can be managed by a simple manoeuvre, by milking the tube underneath from the back forwards after passing urine. It takes a second and it solves the problem.

Sexual dysfunction

This is a big subject. Obviously with so much going on physically and psychologically there can be problems with sex. Chronic fatigue is a simple example – being constantly tired due to being constantly tense doesn't make for a relaxed sex life. A lot of sexual function depends on your autonomic nervous system, similarly to the way your bladder works, so there can be problems with the mechanics of sex. Paradoxically as sex is a very physical, satisfying and relaxing exercise it can be a great consolation to someone who is physically tense all the time.

Fatigue

Chronic fatigue syndrome: we have all suffered from this and know how disturbing it can be. The tiredness is overwhelming and quite unlike the tiredness produced by physical exercise. It is a terrible, oppressive tiredness which is there when you wake up and there when you go to bed.

If you wonder why this happens, do the test. See how tight your neck and shoulder muscles are using the 'thumb test'. What about your tense jaw muscles or the nail marks on the palm of your hand from fist-clenching? If you are sleeping in a tense way, and if you are physically tense all day, no wonder you get physically exhausted. This used to be called 'nervous exhaustion', which is probably a good name for it.

There are other reasons why you can be chronically tired. There is the 'post-viral syndrome', a transient tiredness which comes on after a virus infection like glandular fever or even a severe flu. This can last several months, but someone who has autonomic overload may know what it's like to be chronically tired for a very long time, and may well now guess that this is due to excessive pressure on the nervous system, the autonomic nervous system in this case. Thyroid problems or other medical conditions can cause tiredness, but by far the most common cause is autonomic overload.

In summary

This has been a list of many of the symptoms of autonomic overload. If you combine the physical and the psychological symptoms you can imagine just how disabling it can be. Almost everyone experiences some of these problems at some time in his or her life. It's never fun and it can be frightening. There are other more serious long-term effects which can last a lifetime. We can consider these later in the book, but the presence of such problems makes it extremely important that you get on top of your problems now. The good news is that this book really can help!

6
Some Reasons for Feeling
the Way You Do

So where did your autonomic overload come from? There are many potential answers to this, but a word of warning first – do bear in mind that the answers are not as important as taking action! You can spend hours or weeks going over your past life trying to work it out, but the end goal is to fix the problem. Just understanding why something has developed or looking for something to blame for it will not make it any better. Your key starting point is the fact that your autonomic nervous system is overloaded – and you have to deal with the facts as they are now.

Having said that, as we said earlier, understanding a problem is often the first step in treatment, and many people work more willingly at finding solutions if they have some understanding of the factors underlying the problem. We all like to find the links between cause and effect. Knowing more about why it may have happened can also leave you feeling reassured and less isolated.

Rest assured, then, that your overload didn't come out of the blue – it isn't something you have created, or for which you are responsible. Basically, you were either born with a susceptibility to autonomic overload, which means that it is a constitutional or inherited problem, or else you have learned to be the way you are with the problems you currently have – or a bit of both.

This chapter gives you a list of ideas. Some you will recognize and identify with and some will mean little to you. Some of the answers to these problems lie in this book, some may be more complex and need further investigation. Some might give you ideas and stimulate you to take major steps to change your life. Some might encourage you to seek expert help. As always you are advised to make sure that any help you seek is professional and competent, preferably someone who uses the methods outlined in this book which have been validated by ethical research. There are many charlatans out there.

Overreactive autonomic nervous system

This is the first and perhaps the most important reason for your problems, the one from which others may follow. Quite simply, you were probably born with this. It's in your genes, and the circumstances of your life may have exaggerated the effect. As we've seen already, for some people, the automatic or 'autonomic' arousal of their nervous system happens more easily simply because of their constitutional make-up. They have a 'labile' or 'overreactive' autonomic nervous system, and can no more be blamed for it than for having brown hair, long fingers or blue eyes.

If you can identify with this, remember that it isn't your fault, and you can simply blame your genes. But that isn't the end of the story. There is still much you can do – mostly 'cushioning' or 'dampening' the effect of your overreactive nervous system, which is particularly important for you. Have a look at the later chapters in this book, particularly Chapters 9 and 10, which tell you about relaxation and breathing techniques. We know countless people who have changed their lives by following this advice.

Sensitized autonomic nervous system

Sometimes, you can be born with a perfectly reasonable nervous system, but your life experiences have caused yours to become 'sensitized' and therefore overly reactive to certain situations or to life in general. If you've come through many difficult and stressful times in your young or adult life, or struggled through long-term chronic stress or problems of some kind, your body's nervous system can become a bit like a hair trigger, ready to fire at the slightest touch. Again, this is in no way your fault. You have been a victim of circumstances. But the good news is that you can turn this round, and this book tells you how.

Being bullied or ill-treated as a child, bereavement, illness or divorce, all of this type of life experience is difficult to manage and takes its toll on you. Some experiences you never get over, but for most of us time is a great healer and we do adapt to loss and negative experiences. And do remember that the negative events you have experienced in your life may have been made all the more negative because they have induced autonomic-type symptoms.

But with insight and determination you can build on all of your life experiences and obtain a positive outcome. When you come successfully through a difficult time you will be left with a sense of satisfaction which will help you in the future. There is a silver lining to every cloud, if you can only look hard enough.

Personality traits

People can and do show different aspects of their personality in different situations. Doting father one minute, authoritarian manager the next, indulgent lover the next. And do people not change over time? Angry, moody and stubborn at 18; full of initiative, drive and urgency at 40; cautious, methodical and concerned about the environment at 65.

We are all different from each other and that individuality is something we greatly value – it is to a great extent who we are. If then we are all different, obviously there will be shy people, and forceful people, and all shades in between. If you are shy, sensitive and thoughtful, these can be attractive and valued personality traits – but it's easy to see how they may also make you more vulnerable to overload.

But what if you are out-going and talkative, full of initiative, or quietly confident, and still feel the effects of overload? Perhaps you are in the wrong place at the wrong time. Take the person who loves the company of others and socializes with ease – what if he or she is in a job which involves working alone? Or has to move to the country to look after a mother who has advanced dementia? Or what if you're a perfectionist, and you are in a job where cutbacks mean you just don't have time to do every task in the way you would want?

There are many situations where people can find themselves as the proverbial square peg in a round hole, which can create dissatisfaction and distress enough to make you feel symptoms of autonomic overload.

Take for example a perfectionist like Frances, an office-worker who kept everything neat and tidy and in its place at all times, and couldn't tolerate the slightest untidiness. All was well until a new office junior, Brian, started work, who refused to comply. He said he worked better with a muddle around him. Many of us do. Frances soon found she was losing weight as she had lost her appetite, and her old migraine problem had recurred. She went to see her GP complaining that she just couldn't cope. All the signs and symptoms of autonomic overload.

Not assertive?

On similar lines to personality traits is the often-misunderstood subject of assertiveness. Difficult situations often arise from people not being able to communicate their needs and wishes to others, both at work and in relationships. This is what assertiveness is all about. It is firmly based on the idea that everyone is equal, has the same rights and that in our dealings with other people we should have respect for ourselves and each other. It does not mean being overbearing and aggressive, as is often thought.

By making your behaviour more assertive, you may be able to change a difficult situation into one that can be managed, and prevent other problems from arising at all. Lack of assertiveness can lie at the very heart of many human relationship difficulties and dilemmas, and its effects on an individual can be profound and long-lasting. Making changes can be particularly effective in relationship problems and in the workplace (see Chapter 15 on work).

Previous traumatic experiences

These kinds of experience are of a different order from those mentioned already. If you have had a particularly difficult or abusive childhood or adult relationship, or had other harrowing or distressing life experiences, you can remain very troubled. This can sensitize your autonomic nervous system, as explained already. If you can identify with this, you may find that as well as following the guidance in this book, talking to a specialist counsellor can be particularly helpful.

If you have been involved in a serious motor accident, crime, active military service, or public disaster, you may even experience 'post-traumatic stress disorder', a problem requiring expert professional help. If this should happen to you, don't try to deal with it yourself, seek help through your GP and get it sorted out. If you don't you may find that its effects can be long-lasting. Treated properly, it can be managed.

A *feeling of not having control*

It is important to our well-being that we feel that we have control of our own destiny and our own situation on a day-to-day basis. Good employers will know that allowing employees to exercise control over their sphere of work is vital if they are to function at their best. Constant interference, or a repetitive job with no possibility of having control over day-to-day activities is very difficult to manage and it makes life next to impossible. You need to have some control over your life.

Unfortunately we are increasingly being denied this control. Doctors, teachers and all professionals, as well as shop-floor workers or call-centre workers have the same problem, with decreasing opportunities to use their experience and knowledge. So many of us have to work to 'protocols' now, and this can strip us of our all-important sense of being an independent human being.

Kevin has just begun a course in biochemistry at a large university, and is finding it increasingly difficult to cope with the work. The lectures are complicated, and the pace is faster than he expected. It's difficult to get to know people as the lectures have so many people in them. He now feels after only six weeks that the work is totally out of his control, and that he just isn't up to it. He's also been feeling panicky and light-headed during lectures, and has had to leave the lecture for some fresh air on several occasions. He's sure he'll have to give up at Christmas, and is angry that life isn't fair. Why do these things always happen to him?

Liz is on the same course as Kevin, and has noticed him having to go out of the room during lectures. She found the sudden increase in pace and level a shock at first, but decided she would need to put in more study to keep up, and that seemed to work. She also made a point of talking to other students, and discovered they all felt the same. She finds the library helpful to find books on the parts of the course she finds difficult to understand, and the tutorials are very useful for asking questions. She's confident she can cope with the course and is enjoying the experience.

As early as 1966, J. B. Rotter was describing the significance of people's perception of whether or not they have control over situations. He introduced the concept of 'locus of control', and would describe Kevin as having an 'external locus of control', and Liz, an 'internal locus of control'. That is, Liz feels she has her own, internal control over what happens to her, and that her actions and decisions have an effect on her life experience. So she works harder, finds out how others are feeling, and gets further help from the library. Kevin, on the other hand, feels he has little influence or control over events, and that external factors such as fate or chance are largely responsible for what happens to him. So he sits back and takes whatever happens to him as if he has no power to alter it. A kind of 'learned helplessness'.

Beliefs and control. Rotter's view was that those with an external locus of control are more vulnerable in most situations. Such individuals tend to hold some or all of the following beliefs – what about you?

- Luck and chance play a crucial role in life.
- Success is determined by being in the right place at the right time.
- What happens to us is pre-destined.
- In our lives, we are all subject to forces which we cannot control.
- Most of what happens to us is determined by other people or circumstances.

Of course, in today's world, much of our daily life is unpredictable and outside our control. But just becoming aware that your life is not necessarily subject to the whims of others or to circumstances, and realizing for the first time that you can control your own destiny, that you can make changes, and that you can make choices, can be a most liberating, empowering and revitalizing experience.

A lack of challenge

You may be surprised to learn that lack of stimulus can also stress your system, but it is true. We all need a challenge, or dissatisfaction and sheer boredom can affect us. In a way it's related to some of the things mentioned previously, a feeling of not having control and no outlet for your talents. Call it frustration. You need to be occupied and stimulated mentally if you are to be happy and content, and if you aren't your body will let you know.

It would seem that those who have a sense of commitment, a feeling of control and enjoy challenge, change and new activities are less likely to experience overload. In contrast to this, those who have little personal commitment, feel a lack of control over their lives and enjoy stability rather than change are more at risk. The term 'resilience' has been used to describe a similar concept.

Unhelpful coping strategies

This is normal, and something we have all done. We all have to manage the symptoms we get in the situations in which we get them. The most obvious strategy we use is avoidance. If you are uncomfortable in a situation which you can avoid then you will avoid it. That is a normal response. It may be involuntary, something which you do without really noticing that you do it. It may be very minor, like taking the seat nearest the door, or checking where the nearest exit is. You might use a different corridor or staircase if you want to avoid someone. You might make excuses which convince even yourself, like using the stairs to get fit instead of using the lift – if lifts make you uncomfortable.

You might try not to think about these things, which is difficult unless you are able to blank them out completely. If you have a sore head or neck, other muscle-type pain, diarrhoea or some other symptom, you may medicate yourself, particularly with painkillers, which might make things worse.

Autonomic overactivity can change your behaviour so that you might appear excessively reticent or excessively overbearing, for example being too talkative at meetings, or conversely not speaking up at the right time. These are conscious or unconscious coping strategies. Actively look for such strategies in yourself and try to reduce your reliance on them. Again, look at the later chapters for more suggestions, and especially at Chapters 9 and 10 dealing with relaxation and breathing techniques.

Your lifestyle

Your lifestyle in terms of your routine day-to-day activities can make you more vulnerable to autonomic overload. If you are always on the go, rushing here, rushing there, skipping meals, snacking on fast food, taking little exercise, not getting enough sleep, and making little time for yourself, then your nervous system is on 'high' all the time, and is likely to become stuck there. These and other common lifestyle habits encourage overload, and tackling this will be covered in more detail in a later chapter.

Lack of confidence

When you have to walk into a room of strangers, you wonder why it's so difficult for you, and yet everyone else appears to think nothing of it at all. Or maybe it's having to speak up in a meeting, or go out with friends for the evening. Maybe it's trying to make friends, or find a partner to spend time with. Maybe you just can't seem to get a conversation going when you bump into someone you know in the street, or over lunch with work colleagues. Whatever it is, you wonder why you are so self-conscious while everyone else appears to be so self-confident.

The strange thing is that it is often the person we think is the most confident who is putting on a very effective front and is actually lacking in confidence. Sometimes the noisy extrovert at the work outing is really the person with a crippling lack of confidence who is using this display as a smokescreen to hide behind. Everybody, despite their outward confidence, has doubts and insecurities about themselves. They have just become good at camouflaging these over the years. Or they've become good at only doing the things that they feel confident with.

But sometimes, the shrinking violet in the restaurant, at the party or at work is exactly what they seem to be, someone who desperately wants to improve their confidence in themselves. This book will show you the way.

We've talked about innate lack of confidence, where people can grow up lacking confidence, brought about by childhood experiences or parenting style. But natural confidence can be lost later in life, too, perhaps because of a difficult experience such as an accident or losing a job, or perhaps because of a health problem. Sometimes a mid-life crisis can be to blame, in men or women. People begin to ask themselves what life is all about, and what they've done with their time so far. And they are not happy with the answers and can feel undermined by this. They look around at others of the same age or younger who seem to have achieved so much more than them. Then there are the hormonal and physical changes women are regularly exposed to during their lives, such as pregnancy or the menopause. These can affect a woman's confidence. Bear in mind, though, that confidence can be re-learned, just as it can be lost.

Your attitudes and thinking habits

Confidence in yourself is only one example of a range of attitudes which you may have, which may have been influenced by your previous experiences in life. There are many set ways of thinking about life, others or the world in general which can make you more likely to become overloaded. Here are some examples. Are you sometimes or often:

- particularly suspicious of others
- pessimistic
- prone to feelings of guilt
- withdrawn
- dependent on others
- hostile
- aggressive?

All of these behaviours in the wrong place or at the wrong time can bring with them their own difficulties. Have a think about why you feel or behave this way. Have you evidence to support the way you feel? Is there some other way of looking at things? How would a friend look at it? Who says you should feel this way? Is there another explanation? Question your attitudes, and look for more positive alternatives. They will be there.

'Unhelpful' thinking is a bad habit, and may be an important part of your problem, without you being aware of it. In the same way as questioning your attitudes, remember to analyse the way you think about yourself and about other people, as much as the way you think about the situations you face. Do you use 'ought' and 'should' type thinking? You should get that ironing done now. Your colleague ought to have completed that report by now. Your partner ought to have called you. Who says? Can you be needlessly negative about people, situations or yourself? If you identify with any of these thinking habits, start a new habit of questioning this – every time. Have a look at the advice in Chapter 12 on helpful thinking habits.

Lack of social support

Not having much social support in your life can make you very vulnerable. Without friends, family or a partner to talk to, it can be difficult to cope with the daily hassles, stresses and strains of life, making overload more likely. You may live alone, have moved away from home for the first time, or maybe you're travelling abroad. Your occupation may isolate you. And of course you can be so alone in a noisy crowd.

Living in an unsupportive family or neighbourhood can also leave you vulnerable. You might be living with a partner or a family member who is openly critical, or a friend who keeps telling you that you should 'pull yourself together' or 'get a life'. Maybe you share a flat with others who simply keep themselves to themselves. Or, you could be in an apparently everyday social situation but because of the nature of your character you may not quite fit in, and find yourself isolated.

But whatever your situation, all of us need positive and encouraging social support. This makes life easier to cope with and cushions its problems for us. Those who already have a good support system should make maximum use of it, as an outlet for feelings and as a source of encouragement. You should also accept offers of help, and delegate to others to relieve pressure. No need to feel guilty for doing this.

But if your existing support system could do with some building up, or if you're starting at the beginning and trying to build one for yourself, think about those people who might be supportive to you, and how you could best encourage and make better use of that support. A problem shared really is a problem halved.

Don't attempt to make sudden or significant changes in your life without adequate thought. If any of this does ring true, you might consider how you might want to slowly and carefully change the things that you do in life.

Building up your support system

Here are some suggestions.

- Take it one step at a time.
- Encourage and maintain your existing supportive relationships.

- If someone important doesn't understand, if you think it would help, let them read some of this book to help them to understand better, or try explaining it yourself.
- Create new supportive relationships.
- Get more involved in your community.
- Seek support from an appropriate community organization.
- Join a local social club or other group.
- Consult local directories, libraries or advice centres for suitable support, leisure or social facilities.
- Think about using any support and social facilities at work.

Chronic pressure or stress

We can all experience pressure and stress in our lives but if it is too severe or lasts too long then as sure as night follows day you will get some sort of autonomic symptoms.

That's what it is for – your autonomic nervous system's very purpose is to help your body respond to adverse circumstances. These may be at work (see Chapter 15), or they may be for domestic or financial reasons, or family reasons such as caring for an elderly relative, or bringing up difficult teenagers.

You may understand the reasons for your symptoms very well, but it is hard to do anything about them. Have a look at Chapters 9 and 10 on relaxation, and 12 and 13 on assertiveness and lifestyle. Faced with the demands of a growing family, for example, you may need to stand up for your right to relax, or just ensure you get time to eat a proper meal. Use the techniques we describe later on to help cushion you from stress, including relaxation and breathing exercises. If you can't remove the cause of the stress, take steps to mitigate the effects of the pressure. Do the best you can to make your life easier – and don't feel guilty for doing so.

And so . . .

Remember again, please, that just understanding isn't enough. You now need to move on to the next chapters which contain clear, simple ways to help you change. The next chapters explain how to help you relax, breathe properly and generally cushion or 'damp down' your nervous system so as to make you more comfortable.

7

You and Your Doctor

If we're dealing with a real live nervous system, why can't your trusted family practitioner sort it out for you? What help can you reasonably expect from your doctor, given that many are understandably confused by a condition that has few measurable physical markers and no set treatment?

First and foremost, don't dismiss your doctor in advance. If you have significant symptoms, even if you think that they are due to autonomic overactivity, *do consult your doctor*. Some investigation might be indicated and you should seek authoritative advice. It is possible to suffer from two conditions at the same time and you should be careful not to miss anything. You might need a simple blood test for anaemia or thyroid disease or you might need a little more. If you are older you should have your blood pressure checked. You do have to take care of yourself, particularly if you have autonomic overload. That doesn't mean rushing to the doctor every week, it means being sensible.

If you do visit your doctor, it may help to be assertive (this means communicating clearly, not being aggressive – have a look at Chapter 13 for more on this). This includes having a defined list of symptoms. You might also want to make suggestions about what you think your problem might be on the basis of your observations and what you have read. You might be surprised to discover that your doctor will be pleased to find a patient who will become involved in a discussion about how to proceed. So, use the information in this book to help to make your own diagnosis (remember, it is based on a doctor's own work and life experience of many years' standing). Several hints and tips are included in this book, clues that will help you to come to terms with yourself and your diagnosis. If you help your doctor, your doctor can better help you.

Your doctor's limitations

There are various reasons why your doctor may not be able to help, some of which we have already touched on. The first reason, as explained in Chapter 1, is that this sort of problem doesn't seem to feature very largely in the medical curriculum that is devised and taught largely by hospital specialists.

Second, there is a general misunderstanding in the community of the role of doctors, who seem to be thought of as priests, sex counsellors, public health specialists and just about anything you can imagine. Occasionally, patients have been known to address one of us as 'Father'! But doctors are first and foremost medical scientists. As we've shown, they tend to work in terms of a demonstrable pathology – that is, physical changes that can be measured and treated. This in itself puts limitations on what they can hope to achieve – as we said in Chapter 1.

Third, there are the practicalities. Your doctor may certainly want to help you, but may face real difficulties, such as lack of time. An average appointment is ten minutes. A doctor's most valuable resource is time, and the problem your doctor has in dealing with your condition is that it might take months. Doctors used to get over this difficulty by giving people handouts with some of the instructions and explanations you might find in this book.

Fourth, and perhaps most vitally, a doctor also has a very onerous responsibility. The diagnosis of autonomic overload has traditionally been a 'diagnosis of exclusion'. That is to say that, as there are no signs or tests to establish the diagnosis, all other more serious progressive or possibly life-threatening diseases have to be excluded first. So if you have stomach problems you need a gastroscopy. If you have bowel problems you need a colonoscopy. If you have neck or head pain you may need a scan. All of this is hugely expensive, intrusive and complex and will probably turn out to be negative. Still, in many patients it has to be done. Some kind of elimination may be necessary. All in all, you can see it isn't always easy for your doctor.

Who else can help?

Clinical psychologists or specialist nurses (CPNs) may be available to offer help, advice and support. Other staff members in a medical practice with special training may be able to help you and they might have more time and also the necessary expertise. Ask your doctor who might be appropriate.

There may be self-help groups for people with problems similar to yours, so you could look in the library. These groups may not use the phrase 'autonomic overload', but things like yoga or groups for particular problems you might experience may be available.

Alternative therapists

Alternative therapists offering relaxation or massage may have something to offer, but do beware of the more outlandish and often more expensive forms of treatment. You are in control. You know which aspects of a variable problem may be important for you, so decide which therapy might be appropriate. Are your problems mostly psychological, or are they physical, or are they behavioural? Would life-skills coaching be of value? Would yoga help, or even religion? If you want help, networking, someone to talk to and advise you or just to learn how to relax, then go for that. You don't have to go for anything if you read this book and follow the advice it gives.

Beware of charlatans – as the medical profession deals badly with this problem (and openly admits the fact) there has developed an industry of people offering a list of spurious diagnoses and unlikely treatments. A condition that is simple to understand but difficult to treat can lead to a plethora of confusing diagnoses.

Steer clear of anyone who would take you into the world of the unconventional or the unexplained. There is an explanation for your problems, and it is an honest and understandable explanation. There is no mystery about it, and no need to delve into obscure and expensive pseudo-therapeutic and possibly unsuccessful options. Try the suggestions in this book first. You won't be disappointed.

Treatment options

If we get back to more conventional treatment options, what is there on offer? Mostly of course the best treatment will go along the lines suggested in this book. There is a consensus that this kind of treatment works best.

The preferred medical treatment for chronic fatigue is physical exercise. Don't be offended if your doctor suggests this if fatigue is your main problem, as it often is. Physical exercise can be free;

research has shown it does reduce chronic fatigue, the opposite of what you might expect. There is a difference between what used to be called nervous exhaustion and physical fatigue, and using your body's systems for exercise reduces the experience of autonomic-type fatigue.

Many people expect medication to treat their muscle pain, irritable bowel syndrome, or diarrhoea. Other people might want sleeping tablets or tranquillizers. There may be a place for some of these things in the very short term, but the dangers of reliance on them for very minimal benefit makes them largely unacceptable. Painkillers can make your pain worse and although other drugs like diazepam do relax muscles, dependency is an unacceptable risk.

There is one type of drug that may help. This is the SSRI, a drug of the Prozac type but possibly a new generation of that antidepressant. Prozac itself does help autonomic overload, but there are drugs called paroxetine and citalopram that do the same thing. Again this may be a short-term answer, but if you are *in extremis* this type of medication may be of help to get you started. These drugs are not suitable for young people. And, let's face it, probably most people would rather try other options first. So read on!

8
Making Changes

Understanding your problem, though an excellent start, isn't quite enough. It's time to make a change. The great news is that it is possible to change autonomic overload, and so to change your life.

Already you've come a long way since the beginning of this book and you should now know more about yourself and you should be feeling more optimistic and hopeful. Are you?

You don't have to answer yes. We live in the real world too and we know how difficult it is to deal with the problems we know you have had for years. There have been so many disappointments and reversals, so many unsympathetic people and such a lack of real understanding and help. It is too much to hope that you will now be able to turn things round in one easy step and make things the way you know they should be. What you have to believe and know is that it can and will happen if you want to make it happen.

How ridiculous! Of course you want it to happen! The vision of a world where you are relaxed and comfortable and performing well in every situation is very seductive. No one outside the world of adventure fiction movies (and you know the sorts of people I mean) is so accomplished as to have the luxury of complete confidence and perfect competence in every situation – thank goodness. We all have shortcomings and we all make mistakes. Some of us are tortured by our mistakes, while some of us shrug them off and ignore them. Some of us have to bungie jump in order to experience an adrenaline rush – some of us can get one crossing the road. There are people who dislike their flat autonomic response and lack of excitement, just as there are some of us who regret having too much.

It's a matter of degree. The point is that how you feel is very much a matter of individual temperament, and this chapter explores this idea further. We are all individuals – but fortunately we can all create our own individual roads to change.

The comfort zone

We all like to live in our comfort zone. Some people would appear to do so permanently, apparently relaxed and at ease with themselves all the time. They are few and far between, and if they are comfortable now, they won't be forever because no one is: situations change.

Change is never easy, and we don't promise that it will be for you. So is it worth the effort to change and improve your life? Well, we think so. Why? The answer has to be that, quite literally, you don't know what you are missing. You don't know what your life could be like, or what it might be like in the future. Everyone should take a critical look at their life and see where improvements could be made. Very few people ever do.

However, in the end, it is for *you* to judge whether you should decide to change or not. If you have major problems with confidence, self-esteem, or with your ability to cope with people and situations, then it will certainly be worth the effort because you can make a big difference in all of these areas.

If you just want to perform better at work or in your social life then it is a more difficult judgement to make, but you can still improve the quality of your life and achieve more, so there is much to be gained.

Making the commitment

So it's decision time! If you are going to take the trouble to read this book you might do it just out of interest, but what a waste of time that would be.

You could make a commitment now to work on your problems, and think what the benefits of that might be. So why not just make the commitment now? Know that you can change, you can improve the quality of your life, and resolve that you will do it. Write down or say the words: 'Yes, I will work on my problems, and I will start now.'

You are going to doctor yourself, and that is never easy or straightforward so you need help, either from this book or better from a competent trained person who has a genuine understanding of the problem.

If you have decided to make changes, do take your time. Remember that you didn't get into this situation overnight; indeed, you may have inherited your tendency to autonomic overload from a very early age. Work systematically, making one change at a time after due consideration.

Challenging your assumptions

Athletes know that if they can develop the right psychological approach they can win. If they think they can't win, then they won't. No one ever trains for office work, or for teaching, or whatever. People learn about their job or their life; they learn how to do it, but they assume that they can do it and that their mind and body are in the best possible shape for doing it. But it may not be. Or they may know that it isn't, but believe that there is nothing they can do about it.

Assumptions can form real blocks to change. You may assume, as most people naturally do assume, that your body is working as well as it can. You are the way you are so you just have to get on with it. Why should you assume that? I believe that we can all do better than we do. We are talking about a belief system, an act of faith, and a passion to be the best that we can be.

Self-belief and confidence are key. You know what your intellectual ability is and what you want to and could achieve if you had the right armoury. One of the most frustrating things about autonomic overload is the feeling that you are being held back, almost physically restrained. You just can't do the things you know you should be able to do effortlessly. Anything you do takes a huge amount of effort and courage. You have nothing to be ashamed of; in fact, you probably show courage every day in just doing the ordinary things which some other people may do effortlessly.

Start with the diagnosis

You can't treat something if you don't know what it is. Who is going to make this diagnosis? You're correct, you are! You exhibit extraordinary courage and ability in dealing with your problems on a day-to-day basis; now is the time to redirect that effort into a more productive channel.

The diagnosis laid out in Chapters 4 and 5 on symptoms is much too general for you. You simply can't set about treating all of that. You have to be more specific. You have to know exactly what your situation is, so that you can work out exactly what you have to do to improve it.

Alas, we can't promise you an exciting approach that will be dramatic to use. Your progress will regrettably be slow and rather pedestrian. There is no magic. But, we can promise you an approach that works. So, don't underestimate the advice given in this book. It may sound simple, but you must do it in the way described, in the order it is given, so that you can progress. The strength of character you've already demonstrated just keeping going from day to day – apply this to help you develop habits of thinking, acting and responding which will support you the rest of your life.

Make your database

Let's make a start. What is wrong with you? To be precise, what symptoms do you experience? You may think you know but you don't – not yet, or not precisely. You need *a notebook* for this and for subsequent use. You need to be able to write things down so as to get a clear idea of your problems before you can treat them. In other words you need a diagnosis.

Go back to the list of symptoms and write down in your notebook (or the progress diary at the back of this book) exactly which ones you get, and under which circumstances. Be sure to date this list – you may want to compare it with other lists later on, to monitor your progress. Your symptoms may not be exactly the same as the ones in the list, or they may be slightly different or very different. Start with the obvious and describe them in detail, leaving nothing out. Start with the moment you wake; write down how you feel physically. Then work through a typical day, then through other situations you may experience such as visits to the pub, or shopping. How do you feel? How do you feel beforehand? Do you have diarrhoea? Do you feel sick? Do you feel shaky? Have you had a panic attack? The devil is in the detail, so you need to nail the details.

Now think about the psychological symptoms. When do you feel anxious? When do you feel apprehensive? How do you feel? Describe it if you can't name it. Put the symptoms carefully down the left-hand side and the situations which most provoke them on the right side. Fiddle about with it. You can refine it and make it more accurate over the next few weeks as you begin to notice more. You will notice things in actual situations, things that you didn't know were happening before. If you can, note them at the time, if not as soon afterwards as possible. Keep working on your list until you have made it as accurate as possible.

This list is your database. It is your beginning. It is the start of nailing your ghosts down so that you can deal with them at your leisure. You can add to it or change it. Later we will tell you how to make it more accurate. The more accurate it is the better you will be able to target your efforts.

Extending your database

You are going to check on your symptoms all the time – when you are driving, watching TV, when you are in the pub, at a meeting, in the train or bus. Use your imagination to put yourself into these situations and, if that isn't enough, make a mental or actual note when you are there. What is you autonomic nervous system doing in each of these situations? How overactive is it and what are the results? How much overload do you have?

Scoring your symptoms. The way to nail these problems down individually is to give them a score. This is your next exercise.

You may get the same symptoms in different situations, but they may be more severe in some than in others. Score your symptoms out of 5 (with 5 being the most severe and 1 being the least severe) in each situation on the right-hand side of your list so that you have an accurate record of what you get, where you get it and how bad it is.

Sometimes you just don't feel well, you don't feel right. The problem often is that you haven't identified why you don't feel well. It would be unusual to have a situation where you had general feelings of unwellness coming from your autonomic nervous system overreaction. You would expect to have an identifiable cause such as neck pain or abdominal distension. How do you move from the general to the particular? In the next chapter we will be considering relaxation techniques and you can use these to help identify problems. If you are on a train and feeling unwell, try using relaxation not just to help you to manage your symptoms, but to help you to identify them in the first place. Just sit quietly and relax and check yourself out from head to toe. See what is wrong. You'll find that it helps.

Using your database

If you have been checking yourself out on a regular basis every opportunity you get, as you drive and sit at your desk or whatever, and if you keep a careful record of the way you feel, then you will have acquired a lot of information. You may have had a few surprises. Things that may have seemed easy may not prove to be so, and some difficult things may turn out to be less troublesome than you thought. Don't become too introspective, you are doing this for a reason. You want to become self-conscious.

Now there is a thought! Perhaps you think you are self-conscious enough, and you may be, but here I use the term in its literal sense. You need to become conscious of the way your overloaded autonomic nervous system is working. What is it actually doing to you? What symptoms is it giving you and in what situations do they occur?

Now you have a really valuable, personalized tool that you can use to help yourself. You have a diary, a database, an account of your problem so that it isn't an amorphous mass of misery, it is a list of symptoms unique to you. Having said that, rest assured you're not so different from others. It is often surprising for therapists to see how so many people, each one believing that they have a unique problem, really have much in common.

Setting priorities

After making your database, prioritizing is the next most important thing to do. You can't take on all of your problems at once, no one can. Work out what your worst symptom is and do the same with the situations that you find trigger your autonomic response. A situation is only going to be difficult if you get a severe autonomic response in that situation, so you should be able to make a list. Which problem do you want to tackle? Which problem do you feel might be realistic to tackle? You can't start with your worst problem. You can't start by learning to stand on the stage of a vast auditorium and address a huge audience (unless of course that is the level at which you get symptoms). You are more likely to be symptomatic at a small meeting at work, and certainly that is a situation you will meet more often.

Pick a situation which you encounter frequently and which makes you moderately uncomfortable. It has to be something you can realistically expect to be able to master. That means a situation where your symptoms are not overwhelming, more moderately uncomfortable. Ideally it should be something you experience every day and so can practise every day, such as commuting, shopping, or the school run. Decide that this is the thing which you want to tackle first and determine that you will do just that.

Remember that it may not be a situation which brings on your autonomic overload – it might be a person, or even a thought or an idea. There is another scenario, or it may be a mixture of scenarios. You may have a consistently high level of autonomic activity, in fact you almost certainly will have, but for you it is worse in some situations. Very few people have totally normal autonomic activity most of the time and a very severe reaction in certain situations. It is usually a mixture of the two, and that mix can change depending on your stress levels and the things that are happening in your life. If you do have a severe reaction only in certain situations then you might term this a phobia. Your autonomic response is very focused, but more of that later.

Getting to know yourself

We are almost at the end of our voyage of self-discovery, on the last couple of pages at any rate. You still have the work to do. You should be able to produce a new image of yourself, an image of a competent person held back by problems which are understandable and rational and indeed very common – so common that almost everyone suffers from them from time to time. Finish this paper exercise off by making a note of the things you would like to achieve. I don't mean fanciful ideas, I mean realistic thoughts like having the ability to go to a party without feeling apprehensive or shaky, and to really enjoy yourself.

You will be able to achieve these goals by working on your core problem and applying the general principles to individual situations. Along the way you need to regain your self-confidence and self-esteem so that you absolutely know that you can do the things you want to do in comfort. You need to restore a true image of yourself and see yourself the way you really are. A protracted period of autonomic overload and the symptoms it produces, symptoms like exhaustion, makes you feel that you are incompetent when the opposite is true.

There are many areas we have to investigate, and as we progress through each one we build on the last so that we create a new edifice, one of self-confidence and self-knowledge and a true understanding of the nature of the condition which afflicts us – autonomic overload. Much of the rest of this book is dedicated to a discussion of the ways you can use to help yourself to overcome your problems. Learning about the problem will not make it go away – you have to actually do something about it. The treatment isn't difficult, but it does take time and determination. The rewards are immense, so why pass up the opportunity of changing your life.

The trick is to take on the different elements of your problem and deal with them. There isn't one overriding answer to autonomic overload, no single exercise or way of thinking which will change your life. You have to dissect your problem and reduce it to its elements, and then deal with them one at a time. It is usual to start with muscle tension that is produced by mental tension and over-breathing. You start with the end result, the tension, and you learn to relax that. You do that by a series of relaxing exercises. It sounds simple – simplistic even – but it isn't as easy as it sounds. The results can be very rewarding, particularly for someone who has been physically tense for years. Make a start, you will be surprised by the results.

9

Coping Techniques – Relaxation

You have come a long way to get where you are now. You have considered the nature of the problem in general terms and you should now have a good idea how exactly it affects you personally. What does it do to you? What makes it worse? What is going on in your mind and body?

The chances are that you have been doing the wrong things up to now and you haven't helped yourself. You may have been doing this unconsciously as we all do, reacting to situations and symptoms as they happen and develop.

Go to your own personal symptom list that you have made and recorded in your database. How many of them are due to some element of muscle tension? Headaches, shoulder and neck pain, some types of dizziness and fatigue are all caused by muscle tightness. So let's start our campaign against autonomic overload by dealing with muscle tension.

Dealing with muscle tension

Muscle tension and its associated problems isn't confined to difficult situations. People who suffer from autonomic overload are habitually tense; tension is there in the morning and it can be just as bad at night. It is a habit your body has acquired. Now you have to start to re-educate your body so that you can feel relaxed all, or most, of the time.

We have seen countless people transformed by relaxation exercises. Don't be put off if you've tried these before and had no success. You must have been doing something wrong if you didn't feel at least some benefit. We'll show you the right way to do it here.

I suggest you first try these at a quiet time when you are at your most relaxed, before trying to use them in the situations you have highlighted in your database.

Learning to relax – making a start

Here are three reasons for making an early start and learning this important skill.

- Relaxing is one of the best ways to reduce autonomic arousal.
- Relaxing often also has the added benefit of 'damping down' your body's reactions in the first place.
- Relaxation can help you to pinpoint exactly where your muscle tension problem lies. For example, you might realize that you habitually hold your shoulders tensely, or grip the phone far too tightly, and that you just hadn't been aware of this.

Learning how to relax may not be as easy as you might think. We have worked with many people who have completely forgotten how to relax both their body and their mind, and they have had to relearn it gradually, exactly as we describe below. After all, tension habits may have persisted for years, and may not go away overnight – or even after a few relaxation sessions. Like any skill, such as learning to drive or to play the guitar, learning to relax takes time and practice. Don't worry if you are a little rusty at first – with work and persistence, day by day, it will come. And once it does, you'll never forget how to do it.

Now let's look at some practical relaxation techniques.

Total Relaxation

The idea of these exercises dates back to the 1930s, when Dr E. Jacobson introduced progressive relaxation, which is effective even for severe tension. Allow 20 to 30 minutes for this, and practise every day if you can – at least once, twice if possible. You will need a quiet room where you won't be disturbed. You can either lie down or sit comfortably with your head supported, and ensure you are warm and comfortable, with a blanket or duvet to hand if necessary. If you think you might fall asleep when you relax, make your session earlier in the day.

What you will be doing here is not at all strenuous, but does involve tensing your muscles. Read it through first. As soon as you know what to do, close your eyes while practising, as this is usually much more effective. A few people may actually feel a bit more tense for the first few moments when trying out this kind of technique. Regular practice should quickly sort this out.

Remember! The techniques given here may reduce your alertness and may even make you feel drowsy. While trying out or using any of the relaxation techniques given in this book, and for around 10 minutes afterwards, do not drive, operate machinery, or stand up suddenly. If you are in any doubt about your physical fitness to try this, check with your doctor.

- Lie or sit comfortably, head supported if possible.
- Make a fist and tense up both hands really hard for a few seconds, hold, then let go.
- Slowly repeat this for each of the following parts of your body in turn:

Arms Tighten the muscles in your upper arms and hold that tension before suddenly releasing it. Enjoy the feeling of relaxation and sit quietly for a moment. Slow your breathing down.

Shoulders Do the same thing with your shoulders. Pull them up, hold them up around your ears, hold it, and then suddenly let go. Again rest and enjoy the feeling of relaxation, slowing your breathing.

Neck and head Push your head back to increase tension in your neck. Push your chin slightly forward to increase the tension and then do as above.

Face Frown, tighten your jaw, tighten your face and hold that for a few moments before letting it go, and again enjoy the relaxation. Remember to slow your breathing.

Back and chest You should be getting the hang of it now, but do remember to work slowly and allow pauses between the steps. Arch your back slightly and pull your shoulders down – tighten and hold. And carry on as before.

Tummy Pull your tummy in and hold, count to five and quickly relax, and continue as before.

Legs, feet and toes Rest your heels on the floor and push your toes away from you, but not enough to produce a cramp. Cautiously tighten up your calf muscles and hold as before.

- Once you've completed all the above, remain seated and relax for a few more moments/minutes.
- Rouse yourself gradually. Open your eyes and look around. Slowly stand up and take a few steps. Take what time you need to get back to normal.

This kind of deep relaxation is much like the relaxation you get with self-hypnosis, but don't worry, it is harmless – indeed, essential if you are to combat your autonomic overload. Think of it as a tool, and use it intelligently – when you have practised it for a week or two, you may well find that you don't have to do all the tightening and loosening of muscle groups, and you can drop into this relaxation very quickly. You will then be able to move on to using the faster relaxation techniques below.

Do take your time before moving on. If after a couple of weeks or so you are still finding it fairly difficult to relax using Total Relaxation, then just stick with it for the meantime. It can take time. Some people are more physically tense than others, or have been tense for much longer, so will take more time to loosen up in these circumstances. It's not a race or a competition. Just take this at your pace.

Rapid Relaxation

If you feel that you're relaxing well with Total Relaxation and perhaps becoming a little impatient or bored, then you're ready to move on to one of the faster methods. As before, work on this at least once a day.

Try all three methods given and then choose one which you prefer, or works best for you, to use regularly. If you feel very tense you might like to vary which one you use.

You can still use Total Relaxation whenever you want if you enjoy the longer session. Remember, once you master these methods, you can use them whenever and wherever you want – at home, at your desk, while travelling, or in a meeting.

Technique 1. Lie or sit comfortably, eyes closed, and allow your breathing to become slow and even. Now concentrate on your hands and arms – don't tense them – and concentrate on letting all the tension drain away from them. Continue concentrating like this on each part of your body in turn, as in Total Relaxation:

- hands and arms
- shoulders

- neck and head
- face
- back and stomach
- legs and feet.

Let all the tension drain away, without tensing them first. Enjoy the feeling of relaxation. When you feel ready, finish your session, gradually allowing yourself to become more alert. Have a yawn and a stretch if you feel like it. When you feel alert, return to what you were doing.

Technique 2. Follow the instructions as for Total Relaxation, but speed up the whole process, so that you can become relaxed within a minute or two. Finish off as for Technique 1.

Technique 3. Lie or sit comfortably, allowing your breathing to become slow and regular. Now, all at the same time, tense up your whole body, and hold it tight for a few seconds: hands, arms, shoulders, neck and head, face, back and stomach, legs and feet. Then, suddenly, let it all go, and allow relaxation to take over. Repeat the whole process once more if necessary. Enjoy the relaxation for a few moments or minutes, then finish off your session as for Technique 1.

Why leisure activities may not be enough

At this point, you may be saying, 'But why do I need to learn a special technique to relax? I walk and swim regularly!' Of course you don't necessarily need to use special techniques like these to relax. A walk on the beach, a lazy bath, listening to music, yoga, gardening, physical activity such as swimming or jogging, and so on, can all be relaxing. The key thing is to take time out to do something we enjoy and which is relaxing for us.

For someone with autonomic overload, if you have time, these more simple pastimes might be the first avenue to try. But there can be a number of drawbacks with this everyday approach to relaxation, particularly for a severe or long-lasting problem with muscle tension.

- Arousal and tension may be so persistent that the muscles need to be relaxed frequently, several times a day or more.
- You may be so tense, that this kind of approach just doesn't work.
- Arousal and tension often occur while doing something else, such as in the workplace.
- You may not be able to find an everyday activity which relaxes you.
- Most of these other activities are very time-consuming.

So it often requires more specialist techniques like those given in the exercises above, to get to grips effectively with physical tension.

With practice, many of these techniques can achieve relaxation in as little as a few minutes or, in some cases, even less. So, once you're comfortable with the techniques, experiment. Use them singly or together to suit your individual needs.

Relaxing the mind

So far we've been focusing almost exclusively on relaxing the body. But as you will probably agree, sometimes it's relaxing the mind that is the main problem. Being able to relax physically is an important first step in achieving this, and will go some way to helping your mind to relax. But sometimes a bit more help is needed.

The key point in relaxing the mind is to be aware that simply telling yourself not to think about something or trying to take your mind off your worries won't achieve a thing. The more you try to do this, sometimes the worse it gets. Why? Because the more you do this the more you are actually paying attention to, and concentrating on, your worries. Sometimes they can even grow in your mind and seem much larger than they really are, simply because you keep concentrating on them so much.

The key tip to get your mind off your worries is to give it something else to think about. And the way to make it relax is to give it something relaxing to think about.

So let's give this a try. Lots of suggestions are given here; try them out and see what works best for you. Everyone is different and will find some work better than others. Also, it's a new skill, and like physical relaxation needs a bit of practice. But it's well worth it!

First, use whatever method you have found works best for you to relax your body – either Total or Rapid Relaxation. Then try out the methods given below, and see what works best for you.

Focus 1. Close your eyes and picture in your mind as clearly and in as much detail as you can a calming scene such as:

> waves lapping on the sea-shore
> branches blowing in the breeze
> boats bobbing in the harbour
> corn swaying in the breeze
> dark, deep green velvet.

Focus 2. Focus your mind absolutely on one of these:

> a calming poem,
> a prayer
> a well-loved face
> a well-loved picture.

Focus 3. Repeat silently and very slowly a word or phrase such as:

> r . . . e . . . l . . . a . . . x . . .
> p . . . e . . . a . . . c . . . e . . .
> peaceful . . . and . . . calm . . .
> let tranquillity ease my mind . . .
> so . . . . . . hum . . . . . .
> om . . . namah . . . shivaya . . . . . . (pronounced 'om numaa shivaa-yuh' and means in Sanskrit 'I honour my own inner state')
> other words which you find calming . . .

Focus 4. First, relax your body as much a possible, close your eyes, and try imagining yourself in one of the following settings in as much detail and as vividly as you can:

- By the ocean as the waves roll in . . . and . . . out . . . in . . . and . . . out, feel the spray, hear the sounds, smell the salt in the air . . .
- Relaxing on a fluffy cloud, drifting along and warmed by a shining sun . . .
- On a grassy mountaintop, tropical forest beneath, the morning rains just over, and warmed by the tropical sun . . .

- By a gurgling stream on a warm summer's morning . . . hear the birds singing in the trees and feel the grass beneath your feet . . .

Creative people often find it much easier to imagine scenes or pictures. Words and phrases can be easier for most people. Remember, practice is often required to become good at this, but it can be very helpful in managing your problems. What's important is that you try different methods to come up with something which suits you, and then practise the skill until you become good at it.

Keeping a diary

It isn't enough to learn how to relax in the privacy of your own living-room or bedroom, even though it may make you more comfortable and help you to sleep better. No, you want to take your relaxation out into the outside world, into your car, social events and your place of work. That is the point of learning to relax: to help you get on top of your autonomic overload in challenging situations, when it tends to be at its worst. If you can cope in the worst situation you might have to face you will have nothing more to fear. And 'coping' means getting by, even if it's by the skin of your teeth. If you can know that, your confidence will be restored, you'll cope better each time, and you will never feel you are in the grip of autonomic symptoms again. How do you achieve that?

In addition to your database, a diary is an essential tool. It doesn't matter how, whether it's on a piece of office A4 or in a notebook or as a spreadsheet. Or, you'll find a diary ready to complete in the last chapter of this book.

You have to know what is going on. You have to know when you relax so that you have a record of your backsliding and can do something about it. Take nothing for granted. What works, what doesn't work so well? If something didn't work, why didn't it work? You have to know.

Making a plan

Not necessarily a cunning plan but more of a sensible plan. You need to decide in advance how you are going to deal with problems. For example, do you need to work out strategies for travelling, arriving at work, or going out to a social event? Do you relax at home or in the car or when you arrive? Do you start the day at work with a rapid relaxation exercise? How do you prepare for a meeting?

You don't want to overload yourself further, so make a plan – and keep it simple. Start with one situation which you think you can change. Write it down and record how you get on in your diary, and keep that diary for future reference when you don't think you are making much progress. You can always look back and be surprised, even amazed at what you have achieved without really realizing it.

Keep at it

Really, this is the difficult bit. This is why an adviser, mentor, supportive friend or confidant(e) can be of benefit. You are taking on a great deal, and it is going to be a difficult road to follow. Don't underestimate the difficulties, but don't worry too much either. Remember what you have to gain, and remember how long you have had your problems. Expect slow but demonstrable progress, and expect lapses because it's hard work and you aren't perfect! But do keep at it, and if you lapse, get back to it. The key to success is your determination. But you are going to be a winner, and you will continue to be a winner. So keep at it.

10
Coping Techniques – Breathing

Now we come to one of the most important elements of autonomic overload – breathing disorders. I don't mean major disorders of breathing; quite the reverse. You have probably always assumed that your breathing, which is under the control of your autonomic nervous system, will regulate itself automatically. If you run or exercise, it will speed up and become deeper to maintain the correct oxygen levels in your blood stream. You have assumed that at rest your breathing will be quiet and relaxed. Well, you now know enough about the nature of your autonomic nervous system to know that this isn't automatically the case.

If your breathing is not well enough regulated to keep what doctors call your 'blood gases' in a steady state, within normal limits, then all kinds of problems can develop. These problems aren't serious in the sense that they might be life-threatening, but they are severe enough to cause you symptoms. Many of the most annoying symptoms you get are caused by minor, long-lasting over-breathing – chronic hyperventilation. These problems are so common and so annoying, causing many of the symptoms listed in this book, that we could almost have written the book about hyperventilation alone!

A well-kept secret

Yes, I know, you haven't heard much about hyperventilation before, except possibly in the acute situation where someone becomes hysterical and over-breathes enough to produce tetany, when they develop cramps in their hands and really seem to be very unwell.

But I am talking about a slightly different situation, where your autonomic nervous system speeds up the rate of your breathing just a bit, and also increases the depth of your breathing, so that you alter the transfer of gases in your lungs. You may yawn or sigh more than average while at rest. The resulting alteration in your blood chemistry, though slight, is enough to increase muscle tension, and produce other symptoms. It is the main reason why you get neck and shoulder pain and all the rest.

71

Most people have heard something about adrenaline and the changes it can make, many know about acute hyperventilation, but not so many know anything about this type of chronic hyperventilation. It was first investigated by Professor L. C. Lum in 1977. He was an Emeritus Professor of Respiratory Medicine, not a subject directly related to chronic autonomic problems. He noticed an association between patients with chronic anxiety states (a related problem) and particular breathing patterns. He was able to treat these patients with breathing exercises. His work went largely unnoticed.

However, he was able to show that people with anxiety states, who have high levels of autonomic activity, breathe differently from other subjects. If they can be taught to correct these subconscious, abnormal breathing patterns their symptoms can be controlled. As always with autonomic overload, there is a simple medical logic to explain what happens. In effect, when over-breathing, carbon dioxide is 'blown off' in the exhaled breath, and the blood chemistry is altered. Lactic acid in your muscles, the product of exercise, cannot be neutralized and pain develops. Because the blood chemistry is altered, and your blood goes everywhere, there are many other changes as well, so it's a bit like the release of adrenaline from the adrenal glands – it has an instant effect.

Fortunately this effect can be rapidly changed if you change your breathing patterns. Anaesthetists use inhaled gases because of this potential for rapid reversal. You've probably heard of the situation where the sufferer has to breathe into a paper (not plastic) bag. If someone who has acute hyperventilation breathes into a paper bag, they re-breathe their exhaled carbon dioxide and very rapidly restore their altered blood chemistry, releasing the cramps as if by magic. Chronic hyperventilation takes longer to reverse. It takes longer because it is a subconscious habit.

The test

To see whether you are over-breathing, try this simple test. When you are at rest, for example watching TV, place one hand on your chest and one on your abdomen. You should be breathing with your abdomen only. Watch any sleeping dog or cat.

If you are breathing with your chest muscles you are breathing too deeply. If you are breathing too fast you will know. If you are taking frequent sighs you will notice, or your partner or companion will notice for you.

Dealing with breathing problems

The good news is that you can learn to control your breathing, and make yourself feel better. Now we really have to get down to dealing with this. It's far too important to ignore. It may be the basis of many of your problems. Sorry, there's no magic pill, it's down to you. It isn't difficult, but it takes time and application like all the rest. Don't start to do these exercises until you are comfortable with your progress so far. If you are ready, have a look at these exercises. Do them when you are relaxed, perhaps after a relaxation session.

1–2–3 breathing. Try this out first when you are already fairly relaxed, until you get a feel for it. Practise every day. Then you can use it when you are feeling tense, to help you to feel better.

- Lie or sit with good support.
- Let your breath go, then take a gentle breath in to your own slow silent count of 1 . . . . 2 . . . . 3, and then breathe out again in your own time to your own slow and silent count of 1 . . . . 2 . . . . 3.
- Continue gently breathing to this rhythm for a minute or two.

This sounds simple, and it is – but hundreds of people before you have found it to be very effective at dampening down your autonomic nervous system when it is overloaded. Combine it with your relaxation exercises. You could use a quick relaxation method and then concentrate on your breathing for a few more minutes. Do it often, and at every opportunity until it becomes a habit.

Breathing to relax

As we have seen, one of the most common parts of autonomic overload is persistent hyperventilation, a condition which can silently undermine normal body function and produce a wide range of the symptoms. People can even be frightened by these symptoms and fear major illness. Setting your mind at rest on this score is important.

Persisitent low-level hyperventilation is best relieved through the regular use of breathing exercises designed to re-establish normal breathing rhythms. There are two main approaches to this – sleep-style breathing and alert-style breathing.

Sleep-style breathing. So we've talked about how autonomic overload makes you breathe faster, and mainly with the upper chest. This fills up the lungs, making you feel as if you can't take a breath. When you feel you can't get a breath, quite often it's because your lungs are already full. What you need to do isn't to breathe in – it's to breathe out. The type of breathing experienced in sleep, when we breathe mainly with our tummy or abdomen, can have a very calming effect on you. This can even be used instead of relaxation exercises.

This takes ten minutes now, but when you are used to doing it you can do it for a few minutes, or even seconds.

- Lie or sit with good support.
- Put one hand flat on your navel, the other on your upper chest.
- Let your breath go, then breathe in very gently – notice your tummy rising under your hand.
- In your own time, breathe out again gently, and notice your tummy fall again.
- Continue this gentle breathing, trying to have as little movement of your upper chest as you can.

With practice you will manage to breathe in this way without using your hands, and also when you are standing up.

Alert-style breathing. Other breathing exercises aim to introduce normal breathing patterns with a less calming effect than in sleep-style breathing, and these can be used whenever you need to remain alert, but relaxed. And that's a lot of the time. Many people have found such techniques can be a life-line, as they are so quick and easy to do when needed during a hard day. I've known many people for whom these have transformed their lives.

Try these (we've included 1–2–3 breathing just as a reminder). See which work best for you. Then practise these for a minute or two each day until you can use them whenever you need them to help you to relax and cope better. All can be done unseen whenever you need to relax.

1. Scanning
- Breathe in while silently scanning your body for any tension.
- As you breathe out, relax any tension you found.
- Repeat this breathing in and out several times.

2. Countdown
- Focus on your breathing.
- Count silently backwards from 10 to 0, saying the next number silently each time you breathe out.

3. String puppet
- Let your breath go, then take in a deep breath, hold it for a second or two, then let it go with a sigh of relief, dropping your shoulders and slumping your whole body like a puppet whose strings have been cut.
- Repeat once.

4. 1–2–3 breathing
- Lie or sit with good support.
- Let your breath go, then take a gentle breath in to your own slow silent count of 1 . . . . 2 . . . . 3, then breathe out again in your own time to your own slow and silent count of 1 . . . . 2 . . . . 3.
- Continue gently breathing to this rhythm for a minute or two.

Keeping at it

Use your diary, pen and paper to make sure you work in an organized way and help you decide what works best for you. And, keep at it! That's the most difficult bit. You have to become self-conscious in the literal sense, self-aware. You must keep practising until you are comfortable and relaxed again. You have undertaken the task of learning new habits and 'unlearning' bad habits, and we all know that it isn't easy. Worthwhile things rarely are, but think of the rewards on offer. You'll have a new relaxed life where you will be more successful. Your performance at work and socially will improve, and you will start to look forward to the day, or to your evening out. All you will lose is tension and autonomic arousal, and you have everything to gain.

Remember that this is not a race or a competition to see how quickly you can learn these skills, or how well you can achieve relaxation. No, the main point here is for you to progress at the rate that is right for you. If tension and worrying thoughts have been a big problem for you for a long time, progress may be a bit slower than if you have little physical tension and this has only become a problem recently. So, at your own pace, keep at it. It does work.

From today, what to do

- Practise every day some form of relaxation which relaxes your body.
- Practise every day some form of relaxation which relaxes your mind.
- Practise every day some form of breathing technique.
- When ready, move on to quicker methods of relaxing (if you haven't already done so).
- When ready, begin to use any of these techniques in your everyday life whenever you need them.

11

Coping with Panic Attacks

As you've read, the automatic part of our nervous system is the part that keeps us breathing and our heart beating automatically, without us having to think about it. In our resting state, this system will be ticking over nicely.

But this system can become increasingly aroused. As described already, this is a necessary part of our biological make-up, having evolved in our cave-man and cave-woman ancestors as a self-preservation mechanism, to prepare them to cope physically with whatever situation they might find themselves in, especially a dangerous or threatening one.

So in the case of an approaching snarling sabre-toothed tiger, instant autonomic arousal prepared cave men to either 'fight' the animal, or 'flee' as fast as they could. This all happens extremely quickly and completely automatically, because if our ancestors had taken time to think about it, it would have been too late! Every split second counted in our early days. So we breathe faster, think faster, our heart beats faster, our muscles become taught and ready for action, our blood-sugar levels rise to give rapid energy, increased amounts of adrenalin are produced, and so on. All this to prepare us for instant and effective action.

But in the huge time-span that is human evolution, our cave-dwelling days were relatively recent, so our bodies are still reacting in exactly the same way today. But with a twist. This reaction developed as a primitive response to physical danger, such as the infamous sabre-toothed tiger. But today, it is just as easily brought into play in our high-speed world, by psychological danger. In other words, when there is danger to us as a person. For example when we are afraid of losing face, or not being able to cope, or being embarrassed in public, or if we feel out of control of our lives.

However, in our modern world, we can't fight with our line manager, or run away from our debts, much as we might want to. So in today's world there is seldom a physical outlet for the ancient fight-or-flight reaction, and the arousal it produces. All those major bodily changes are still there, but have no outlet, leaving you feeling very strange indeed. Ready and able to fight that tiger, but in reality sitting at your desk, desperately trying to figure out why your computer has crashed for the third time today, or in a very long supermarket queue, panicking about how you're going to get home in time. This is when panic can strike. Your stomach may churn, heart race, breathing may be rapid, and you may sweat, feel faint, feel overwhelming fear and panic, and a sense of impending disaster, along with a pressing need to escape from the situation you find yourself in. It's a distressing and very frightening way to feel: a full-blown panic or anxiety attack.

As you know, this panic response is often triggered by events, but it can even by brought on by something as transient and unsubstantial as a fleeting thought in your tired mind, especially with a sensitized nervous system. 'What if I can't get this done in time?' 'What if I can't pay those bills?' 'What's my boss going to say?'

Understanding what is happening to you and how to deal with it, can diffuse a situation. If nothing is done about it, you can surprisingly quickly find yourself beginning to avoid situations you feel you may panic in, like shops, restaurants, work, visiting friends or the pub.

A panic attack like this can be very frightening. You may well know this first hand. It feels like being the victim of a terrifying attack over which you appear to have absolutely no control. You can be convinced that you are going mad or are about to faint or die.

If you don't regain control over these attacks which seem to strike out of the blue, a vicious circle can quickly, if not immediately, establish itself. Still higher levels of arousal will be produced as you worry about the next attack, and avoidance behaviour will be targeted on the situations which you fear may provoke another attack. The fleeting thought, 'What if I panic now?', can immediately set off the feared attack. It becomes alarmingly easy then for a serious phobia to rapidly develop due to avoidance. So what can you do if you have panic attacks?

Four tactics against panic

1 As described already, your level of anxiety and arousal is often substantially reduced simply by understanding the bodily processes which make you feel the way you do. This is even more true for panic attacks. Once the fight-or-flight reaction has been

explained and understood, the fantasy of an unpredictable and terrifying attack can be transformed into the reality of a completely natural and ancient automatic defence mechanism as we've described already. This can have a rapid and remarkable effect on you.

Margaret was suffering from panic attacks, and attended a seminar run by a local voluntary group. So unsteady was she that she required physical support to reach her seat to listen to an explanation of panic attacks being given by a clinical psychologist. She sat shaking at the back next to the door, hardly able to speak for anxiety. Yet by the end of the explanation she was in the front row confidently asking questions. The difference was she now understood what was happening to her physiologically.

2 Reduce your stress levels as much as you can, by removing or reducing any stressors in your life. This reduces your risk of having a panic attack.
3 Cushion or dampen your nervous system as much as possible using the full range of techniques discussed in this book. These strategies will also make panic attacks much less likely to happen to you.
4 Learn to notice the first signs of a panic attack beginning, and use a quick relaxation or breathing technique at that point, to prevent the panic attack progressing any further. As the panic response is an automatic process, like breathing, simply telling your body not to panic will not be effective. Physical relaxation techniques on the other hand, can reach behind the automatic response, allowing the brain to realize that the danger is subsiding, and begin to press the 'no need to panic' button. The PAUSE routine, which we explain next, describes clearly how to do this.

Coping with a panic attack – the PAUSE routine

'We have nothing to fear but fear itself,' as Franklin D. Roosevelt said. So, if you have panic attacks, the key is to catch them early, and stop them in their tracks. This puts you back in control. Here is one way of doing this. Don't be put off if this method doesn't work the first or even second time you try it. Keep at it. It takes a bit of practice, and a bit of determination, but it is very effective. Thousands of people have used it successfully. You can too.

First, work out what are your own first signs of a panic attack. This might be a lurch in the stomach, a thought in your mind, heart rate rising, or something else you've noticed. Be on the lookout for these first signs. When you notice them, you should immediately:

Pause ... and make yourself comfortable (sit down, lean on something etc.).

Absorb ... detail of what's going on around you.

Use ... any method of relaxing quickly which works well for you, then

Slowly ... when you feel better,

Ease ... yourself back into what you were doing.

If you've been practising quick ways of relaxing, now is when it pays off big-time. When using the PAUSE routine, you can use whichever of these methods has worked best for you – be it rapid relaxation, a breathing technique, or any combination you've found useful.

12
Helpful Thinking

We all know people who remain positive and unbowed in the face of difficult circumstances, and others who simply crumple and give up hope. Look at Christopher Reeve, who never gave up fighting his major disability, and campaigning to help others right up until his untimely death. On the other hand, we probably all know someone in our family, or in our own street, who finds the smallest difficulty enough to make them throw in the towel. The difference lies quite simply in how these individuals think about their situation. The difference is in their attitude to life – how they think about it, and how they assess their ability to cope with it. Most of us fit somewhere between these two very different extremes. Where do you think you might fit in?

Of course, our judgement of each situation we find ourselves in, and our ability to cope with it, can have a major impact on whether we experience autonomic arousal or not. Indeed, how we think about the world in general, and our own world in particular, can even be causing us a problem in the first place, and producing autonomic overload.

How we think about our world can affect us in two distinct ways:

- It determines our reaction to a problem situation – be crushed by it, or take it in our stride, or somewhere in between. So it's not just about the situations we find ourselves in – it's about our attitude towards that situation, and our ability to cope with it.
- Our thinking can actually be the cause of our feeling pressured or discontented in the first place – for example, expecting too much of ourselves, expecting too much of other people . . .

Thinking habits and beliefs

We are not talking here about the kind of thinking which could be considered wrong or as an illness of any kind. No, I just mean normal everyday patterns of thought and belief that encourage us to react adversely to the things that go on in our lives. Our thinking habits are largely established during our childhood, often copied from our parents. But they can also be a response to the experiences we've had in our lives. Some of our thinking patterns and habits will be substantially influenced by our cultural background.

You may be surprised to hear that the way we think is not fixed for life. It can be changed. So you will be asking, what can you do to change your thinking? This chapter will explain how you can do just that. To start us on this remarkable journey through our thinking processes, I have to go back to the 1960s when this whole idea of helpful and unhelpful thinking began to grow and develop, and ways in which you might alter your thinking for the better had been established. The general idea was that you first had to become aware of the thinking styles and beliefs that might be causing you a problem, and then think of ways to change these for the better. For many people, just becoming aware of their established patterns of thought, along with the detrimental effects these could be having, can be enough to bring about a substantial, effective and long-lasting change.

To anyone not familiar with such ideas, they may seem unusual. But in my experience most people find these surprisingly effective. You may too. Here's a bit more detail.

Unhelpful beliefs and how to challenge them

In 1962, Dr Albert Ellis began to explain how problems can arise out of the beliefs we hold about the world. He described these as unhelpful beliefs in the sense that they are inflexible and dogmatic. But don't worry, they don't in any way represent a problem or an illness. Such beliefs are extremely common and can be seen as entirely 'normal'.

Here are a few taken from an extensive list of examples. Are you able to see how holding even one of these beliefs can make life difficult?

- Life should be fair.
- I should be able to do everything well.
- There should be a perfect solution for everything.
- I need everyone's approval for nearly everything I do.
- I should not make a mistake.

Most of this thinking is a direct result of growing up and living in a world where performance standards are set high, praise for a job well done is seen as encouraging an undesirable swollen head, and criticism of mistakes is never far away. For many of us, this has produced low self-esteem, lack of confidence and fear of failure. If this strikes a chord with you, you must become aware of and challenge these beliefs. This should mean that their capacity for causing problems will be reduced.

So, to begin with, understand that these beliefs are not undisputed truth. No, they have their roots in childhood, life experiences and the culture around us. If you have any of these beliefs, you should ask yourself where these beliefs are written down or stated. Who says?

Here is the same set of unhelpful or mistaken beliefs, along with ways of challenging them:

- Life should be fair. (Who says? How could it possibly be?)
- I should be able to do everything well. (Who says? Do you know anyone else who can?)
- There should be a perfect solution for everything. (Who says? How could there be?)
- I need everyone's approval for nearly everything I do. (Why? Who says? Is it possible anyway? You can't please all the people all the time.)
- I should not make a mistake. (Do you know anyone who doesn't make lots of them?)

Many unhelpful beliefs include the words 'ought', 'should' or 'must' – use of this last one is often described as 'musterbation':

- I ought to have done that better. (Why? Who says?)
- I must cope with everything. (Why? Who says?)
- I should have done that better. (Why? Who says?)
- I must not make a mistake. (Everyone does – why can't you?)
- I must get all this done today. (Why? Who says?)

Other beliefs and thoughts involve the words 'awful', 'terrible' or 'can't stand it', which usually exaggerate the reality of the situation:

- I can't stand this. (You've stood things like this before, you can do it again, is it really as bad as all that?)

- This is absolutely awful/terrible. (Some things are, but is this? What words have you left to use if something even worse happens?)

Wendy recently came to see me. She was in her 30s, and looked tired, pale and desperate. She told me her story.

'I feel under pressure all the time. I just can't understand it. We have a lovely house, two beautiful children, and I have a good relationship with my husband, Geoff.'

When I asked her to describe her usual day, she said:

'Let me see, now. I must get the shopping and housework done before lunch-time, so that I can get to work on time at one o'clock. I must leave the house tidy, so that I don't have to tidy it when I get back. I have this absolutely awful job at the supermarket, stacking shelves. I can't stand it, but we need the money. Then I rush home to cook dinner. I really ought to do more home cooking and baking for the family but trying to fit everything in is so terribly difficult. It isn't fair really, I try so hard, but I never seem to get it right. There must be some easy answer to it all, because everybody else seems to cope better than I do.'

Can you see how much of Wendy's thinking is causing her unnecessary pressure? She sets rules and expectations for herself which are impossible to meet, exaggerates situations, and is angry with life because it doesn't all work out the way she wants. It is quite common for much of this type of thinking to interlock together in a kind of 'ideology of life'.

It's not that Wendy deliberately thinks in this way, and is responsible for her difficulties. These are simply thinking habits and beliefs that can creep up on many people in today's hectic world where success, possessions and coping are so valued. It is very common indeed.

Thinking more positively

Are you aware of the constant conversation you have with yourself, silently, inside your head? Donald Meichenbaum has developed techniques based on the idea that this conversation or 'self-speech' exerts considerable control over what we say and do. Think about it. What sort of conversation goes on in your head every day? Be honest. Do you have a negative style of self-speech? Can your inner dialogue be self-defeating and discouraging? This can aggravate low self-esteem.

Do you ever have thoughts such as:

- I'll never manage this.
- I'm hopeless at this.
- I can't do anything properly.
- Oh no, here we go again.
- This is going to be really difficult, I don't think I can cope with it.

Like unhelpful thinking habits, this inner speech is seen as a habit which can be changed. Once aware of this inner self-defeating speech, you would be encouraged to use other truthful but realistic phrases such as:

- I've coped with this before, so I can do it again.
- I know I can do this if I really try.
- I know I can do this quite well, and that should be good enough.
- Everybody makes mistakes and so can I.

Thinking distortions in close relationships

Aaron Beck is another eminent figure who believes that our thinking can affect us in ways we hadn't envisaged. He has produced a great deal of work on this general subject, and among this he has described some of the common thinking distortions to be found within most marriages or close relationships. Do you recognize any of these?

Magnification: The tendency to exaggerate your partner's less attractive traits.
Polarized thinking: All or nothing, right or wrong, or black-and-white thinking, with nothing in between.
Negatively biased thinking: Making quick and negative judgements and conclusions, without evidence.
Tunnel vision: Tendency to focus on one comment or detail and blow it up out of proportion.

Gaining a sense of control

Control is a theme which has run through much of this book, and we return to it here. People vary in the extent to which they feel they can affect their situation, or that they have some control over what happens to them.

People with what is described as an 'external locus of control' feel they have very little control over their lives. 'Locus' just means where the control centre is. Such people will believe that what happens to them is all down to other people and to the situations they find themselves in. Because of this, they will probably have taken none of the available steps to help themselves to cope better. They may even consult astrologers or clairvoyants to find out what lies ahead for them.

Other people, who have what is called an 'internal locus of control', feel that their control centre lies within themselves. In other words, they don't feel at the mercy of outside influences. They feel they have control over their lives, and they use that control to cope and to make changes for the better.

Which category do you think you fit into? Do you have an 'external' or 'internal' locus of control? Where is your control centre?

This idea might even partly explain the crucial difference between people who crumple and those who flourish when faced with adversity. The former sees the situation as beyond their control and gives up, while the latter takes control and takes the required action to turn the situation around and make it manageable.

If you feel you can do nothing to affect your life and your situation, you need encouragement to change your mind and to take action, to make your life better and more fulfilling. That's what this book is trying to give you.

Some general hints and tips for helpful thinking

- Don't ignore the ordinary or good things that happen each day, as if they don't count for some reason. Take account of the bad side, but don't dwell on it.
- Take your mind off your problems as much as you can – they grow bigger the more you concentrate on them, but shrink into proportion when you think about something else.

- Remember that when things go wrong it's not always your fault – other people or simply the situation are just as likely to be to blame.
- Get into the habit of thinking a positive thought frequently throughout the day – 'What a lovely blue sky', or 'Thank goodness I don't need to go out in that rain'. Your thoughts are up to you, but keep them coming! It may sound silly, but it really works.
- You probably find some thoughts often slip into your mind like, 'I can't cope', 'I'm no good at this'. When this happens, challenge these thoughts. What evidence is there to support these thoughts – and what about the evidence against them? How would others view the situation? What would you say to a friend who felt that way?
- Grow to like yourself. There will never be anyone else quite like you.
- Remember that many people, despite how they appear, are often as unsure of themselves as you are.
- Don't take part in 'negative conversation'. Change the subject to something more positive.
- Encourage friendships with people who have positive thinking habits.
- Don't carry the world around on your shoulders. Give everybody else a share!
- Practise liking people.
- Count your blessings – old-fashioned, but true.
- Avoid jumping to conclusions. We sometimes make decisions (usually wrongly) about a situation with no real evidence to support it, for example deciding a new friend doesn't like you because they refuse an invitation from you (when they probably have a valid reason for doing so). So, weigh up all the evidence before reaching decisions.
- Sometimes we impose high standards or 'personal rules' that produce frequent thoughts containing the words 'should' or 'must' or 'ought', for example 'I ought to do that ironing now', or, 'I must reply to that letter today'. The standard is often set extremely high, and you impose stress on yourself because of it. Ask yourself who is setting these 'personal rules' and whether they are of too high a standard. Let yourself off the hook, and lower those standards if necessary.

And lastly – a plan of action

If you have identified any 'unhelpful' thinking habits you might have, after reading this chapter, go back and underline or highlight these for future reference. Being aware of these really is half the battle.

A little bit at a time, try out some of the advice given but, as usual, don't rush at it – a life-time's habits take time to change.

Refer back to this chapter every so often to remind yourself of the various ideas, and to check out how things are changing in your thinking. Use your diary to help you if you want.

13
Assertiveness

As mentioned already, the idea of assertiveness is based on the idea that everyone is equal, has the same rights and that we should have respect for ourselves and for each other. Many people confuse assertiveness with aggression, but nothing could be further from the truth.

Assertiveness is about being able to express your needs and views in a calm, confident manner that respects both you and the other person involved. Sounds easy when I put it like that. But how do you manage this?

Let's start by taking a look at some general examples of people who are not being assertive, and who are likely to encourage problems for themselves, or for the people they interact with. Do you recognize yourself, or maybe somebody you know? People who:

- find they cannot say 'no'
- cannot speak up about their own needs to others
- are overbearing, rude or aggressive to others
- get their own way by making others feel guilty
- cannot give criticism without devaluing the other person
- have to win at all costs
- can't make up their minds
- manipulate you to get what they want
- use sarcasm
- use 'put-downs'
- don't listen to your point of view or what you have to say.

This type of poor interpersonal communication, whether at work, home or elsewhere, is clearly going to cause problems for those involved. It will affect all relationships from the most intimate to the most public. Improving assertiveness skills can change a difficult or impossible situation into a more manageable one.

So much for generalizations, but what exactly is assertiveness? How does an assertive person behave? This is sometimes difficult to pin down, but here are some pointers to what assertiveness involves:

- knowing your own needs
- being aware of and acknowledging your own strengths and weaknesses
- having genuine respect for yourself
- having genuine respect for others
- being open, direct and honest whenever appropriate
- being able to compromise.

Sounds simple, doesn't it? But it can be very difficult to achieve in the real world, especially if you have baggage from the past which undermines your image of yourself.

Non-assertive behaviour

Let's look more closely at the kind of behaviour which is not assertive. The most common is a package of behaviour such as apologizing for yourself, not standing up for yourself, and an inability to say 'no' to people. This is called *passive* behaviour. On the other hand, this kind of behaviour can show itself as an overcompensating abundance of confidence or humour, which the person can hide behind.

Sometimes the inner frustration of it all can come out as intimidating or *aggressive* behaviour. Shouting, rudeness, anger, lack of tolerance, and even physical violence. There can also be the normally passive person who suddenly and explosively has had enough, and out it can all come in an angry or even violent outburst – no doubt followed by a bout of apologizing.

But all of these various non-assertive behaviours make life more difficult for us. If we don't tell people what we want, we certainly won't get it. If we come over as too confident or aggressive, we'll find work and relationships fraught and unrewarding. If we are persistently passive in our behaviour, this can simply stoke the boiler of resentment until it explodes at a later date – causing even more problems.

Here are the four most common examples of non-assertive behaviour:

Aggressive: angry, in-your-face, verbally abusive, threatening, domineering, competitive, dogmatic, must have your own way, must win, must be right . . .

Manipulative (or indirect aggression): getting your own way by making others feel guilty, by sulking, by sarcasm and put-downs . . .

Over-confident: nothing's a problem, loud, you know best, full of ideas, you know everything, one-upmanship, you know every-one . . .

Passive: dropping hints, making excuses, unable to say 'no', the dogsbody, difficulty making decisions, apologizing all the time, putting everyone else first all the time . . .

Rate yourself

How assertive do you feel you are generally? Before you begin the next activity, rate yourself on a scale of 0–70, where 0 means never assertive and 70 means assertive all of the time. Think about it for a second or two, and write your score down somewhere on a piece of paper. Indeed you might like to repeat this activity say once a month, so you can monitor your progress.

Assertiveness questionnaire

A short questionnaire can give you a feeling for your own level of assertiveness. This is in no way an actual measure, it's simply designed to give you a flavour for the idea. You can take it further if you want to, by reading up on the subject, or taking a course in your own area.

Rate whether you agree or disagree with each statement on a scale of 1–7, and enter the number in Column 1.

1 = strongly agree
2 = moderately agree
3 = slightly agree
4 = neither agree nor disagree
5 = slightly disagree
6 = moderately disagree
7 = strongly disagree

Assertiveness questionnaire

Statement	Column 1	Column 2
I have difficulty saying 'no' to people.		
I often give in to other people's wishes and set aside my own.		
I find being criticized difficult.		
I am prone to aggressive outbursts.		
I feel much better about myself if I please other people.		
I find saying what I really think difficult.		
I often think other people are more important than I am.		
I say 'I'm sorry' a lot.		
I often get my way by making others feel guilty.		
I find speaking up in a group difficult.		
TOTAL SCORE		

As a rough guide, scores of 60–70 indicate you are almost always assertive, 50–59 you are assertive most of the time, 40–49 assertive some of the time, 20–39 assertive occasionally, 0–19 hardly ever or never assertive. How does your score compare with your own assessment above?

Now choose someone you know well – a friend, a partner, or a colleague perhaps. Don't write down their name, but repeat the questionnaire, rating them in your view, for each statement, in Column 2. Total it up. This may or may not reveal interesting differences!

So, having thought about assertiveness, and what it is, let's return to the other sorts of behaviour, those which are the alternatives to being assertive. Of course, we can all behave in each of these ways sometimes. What we should be aiming for is to increase the number of times we are assertive. We can all have off days!

Emily had one daughter and two grandchildren, of whom she was very fond. Though she had a very tiring part-time job in a florist's, she loved to look after the two girls, aged four and seven, when she could. But then her daughter started taking her for granted, assuming she would take care of the girls, often with no notice and even if Emily had other plans – and Emily just couldn't say no. Emily also did shopping and housework for an elderly neighbour, even though he had family of his own. Small wonder if Emily began feeling completely drained, very tense, and starting at the slightest noise. She just couldn't seem to relax, and developed pain in her shoulders and neck.

Paul worked in a large high street shop and had just been promoted, with supervision of several sales assistants. He was finding it stressful because none of the assistants seemed to like him, and appeared to go out of their way to annoy him. He felt agitated and couldn't think what he had done to upset them, though he suspected it might be the way he evaluated their actions. He found it hard to criticize in a way that didn't come across as devaluing them, and hence resulted in their angry feelings.

Emily just couldn't say no, and needed to learn how to do so in order to take control of her workload. Paul needed to learn how to criticize constructively, and with respect, to regain his colleagues' respect and his own former enjoyment of his work.

Everyone's behaviour will vary from situation to situation, but if a lot of what we do is not assertive, this can cause autonomic arousal, and in time overload. Remember, our behaviour varies from situation to situation. You might be manipulative with your partner, passive at work, and aggressive with door-to-door sales-people. So what can you do?

How to be more assertive

Take this slowly and gradually, and try out one new thing at a time. If you find these ideas particularly helpful, remember, you could think about enrolling for a full course, or read up on the subject.

Tick or underline any of these you might find helpful.

- Work out your priorities in life; choose them for yourself.
- Don't try to do everything.
- Make use of your right to choose (and other rights, see below).
- Value yourself.
- Value other people.
- Work out what you need and want in life.
- But be prepared to compromise over these and over other situations which arise.
- Keep to any point you're making – don't let others distract you.
- You cannot be assertive if you are angry – so work off the anger before you deal with a situation (see below).
- Keep your voice slow, steady and low-pitched, and stay relaxed.
- Keep your head up, use regular eye contact and confident posture.
- Get your feeling of self-worth from within yourself, not just from other people.
- Avoid losing your temper and acting aggressively (see below).
- Avoid being too timid.
- Don't expect your obliging ways to prompt others to confirm your value as a person. Get your feeling of self-worth from within yourself, and get to like yourself. Remember nobody's perfect, neither you nor other people!

Saying 'No'
- Keep it short, and say it confidently and warmly.
- Only give a reason if you want to.
- Use a simple phrase you're comfortable with, such as 'I don't want to', or 'I'd rather not'.
- Calmly repeat your 'No' if the first one is not accepted.

Remember you have these rights:

- to make a mistake;
- to have your own point of view;
- to fail if you try something;
- to try again;
- to expect others to listen to you;
- to feel anxious at first.

Deal with your anger when you're alone by:

- punching a pillow, cushion, bed . . . anything soft that you won't damage;
- tearing up old newspapers;
- taking a deep breath and yelling 'I hate everyone!' Then take another deep breath and let it out with a quiet 'Now I feel better and I'm ready to like people again';
- stamping your feet and shouting your angry feelings out loud (when you're alone!);
- taking up a contact sport such as football or judo if you're fit – this can be a great release;
- writing down your angry feelings, then tearing them up!

Even if it's just these hints and tips that you're going to try out, remember you should:

- put any new behaviour or techniques into practice slowly and carefully;
- start with 'easy' situations to develop your confidence;
- then work slowly towards more difficult situations;
- slowly, carefully and step by step, build your confidence as you go;
- don't feel that you have to make big changes . . . it's all up to you.

And always remember, assertiveness is not about being aggressive, it is simply about being able to express your needs and views in a calm, effective manner in a way that respects both you and the other person/s involved. Sometimes all you need is the confidence in yourself to do just that.

14

Changing Your lifestyle

What do you do on a Tuesday morning, on a Thursday afternoon, or at weekends? Where are you to be found on a Friday evening? We all have a schedule of some kind, be it organized or ad hoc and spur of the moment. What is your favourite food? What do you do for entertainment? Where do you go on holiday? We all answer these questions very differently, because we all have our own lifestyle, and a set of day-to-day activities to go with it.

But what you are doing with your time, and the sorts of activities you get involved in day to day, and week on week, can either be making you more vulnerable to autonomic overload or cushioning you from it. Let's see if we can work out which it is likely to be doing for you.

Activity questionnaire

Circle your answer to each question

Do you drink less than 3 cups of coffee or tea a day?	YES	NO
Do you eat breakfast most days?	YES	NO
Do you usually take your time when eating meals?	YES	NO
Do you eat healthily most days?	YES	NO
Is your weight in the 'normal' range?	YES	NO
Do you take exercise most weeks?	YES	NO

Do you almost always have time for lunch and other breaks?	YES	NO
Do you have week-long breaks at least twice a year?	YES	NO
Are you content with how much is going on in your life?	YES	NO
Do you feel you regularly have someone to talk to and share things with?	YES	NO
Do you take part regularly in a leisure pursuit or hobby?	YES	NO
Do you feel you usually get enough sleep?	YES	NO
Is your alcohol intake within recommended levels?	YES	NO

I'm sure you will have worked out that for maximum cushioning from autonomic overload, a YES answer for each question would be preferable. However, we do live in the real world, so most people will circle NO at least a few times, with others ranging upwards from there.

The essential point is that the more times NO is chosen in questionnaires of this kind the less an individual is cushioned, and the more likely it is that they may have difficulties coping with any problems that arise. Indeed, a large number of NO answers may be a cause of problems in itself. For example, rushing meals, not taking breaks and not getting enough sleep will make life pressured and difficult anyway. Don't underestimate such factors as a cause of your overload.

So, a vital aspect of reducing your autonomic arousal is to look at your lifestyle in terms of:

- diet
- exercise
- leisure time
- sleep
- time management
- intake of alcohol (or other drugs)
- social support.

Lifestyle changes that people tend to slip into naturally when under pressure often simply make matters worse: working too hard, for too many hours, not taking breaks, eating too quickly, drinking too much, or skipping meals altogether, to name but a few. Best to make only one change at a time, using a simple diary like the one given at the end of this book, to keep tabs on progress and to plan the next step.

Lifestyle points to target

Here are some of the main strategies for cushioning that are associated with our everyday lifestyle. Tick, highlight or underline those you may find particularly helpful.

Eating. Eat a healthy well-balanced diet, low in sugar, salt and fat, and high in fibre. In particular for cushioning against autonomic overload, eat a good breakfast, don't skip lunch, and avoid sugary snacks or long gaps (two to three hours at most) without eating. This ensures a constant blood-sugar level which helps to protect you from overload. Don't drink too much coffee or other drink containing caffeine (e.g. cola).

Time management. Most importantly, if you feel pressurized in a situation at work or home, make sure you take regular breaks from it. No matter how busy you are, a break will refresh you, put things into perspective, and allow you to carry on more efficiently. Taking regular breaks allows arousal to be reduced regularly, and will gradually diminish the overall sensitivity of your nervous system.

This principle operates at several levels. A ten-minute break every morning, a day out at the weekend, or two weeks on holiday in the summer all help to inhibit overload all year round.

If your life revolves around others most of the time, make sure that you take some time for yourself, and to be yourself. It really is OK to take time for yourself! Conversely, if you have too much time on your hands, involve yourself in voluntary work, hobbies, clubs and so on, preferably with other people. If you find time is very tight, with far too much to do, try some of these:

- keep lists of jobs to be done;
- select and prioritize what you do;
- plan activities – daily, weekly, monthly;
- keep a diary;
- delegate jobs to others;
- do one job at a time, not three or four;
- be organized – know where everything is.

Leisure. Whatever your circumstances, make sure you do things you enjoy on a regular basis – this acts as an excellent cushion. Leisure pursuits can also provide support through the friendships they can bring, reduce pressure by giving you a break, give you something to do if you have too much time on your hands, or provide a new challenge if you need one.

Leisure pursuits help to prevent your identity and self-image relying entirely on a difficult situation such as at work or at home. Make sure you have a good balance between 'work' and 'home' or leisure activities – your 'work–life' balance.

Exercise. Not only is this generally good for you, but physical activity has an excellent cushioning effect, and can allow you to use up feelings of anger and frustration safely.

The keys to effective exercise are:

- finding an exercise or activity which you enjoy and which fits in with your lifestyle;
- doing it regularly.

Always check with your doctor if you're unsure about your fitness with regard to starting or resuming an exercise or activity routine – though walking is generally OK for most people.

Sleep. Getting enough sleep is vitally important to refresh your body and brain. If getting to sleep is a problem, make sure you take regular exercise (see above) as this will help. Any form of relaxation or breathing exercise will help you go to sleep, or get back to sleep if you wake up during the night. An overactive mind, a common cause of insomnia, can be calmed with the methods already given in a previous chapter.

Using some form of relaxation of mind and body immediately before sleep will improve the restful quality of your sleep. It will also be much more refreshing.

If you find you are very sleepy, and sleep too much, the same advice applies. Physical activity during the day, teamed with lots of relaxation of mind and body, especially before your night's sleep, will give you much more productive sleep, refreshing and reviving you much more than dozing off all day.

One change at a time

Making changes in some or all of these areas will improve the cushioning effect of your lifestyle and form an important and long-term part of the new you. That said, again, making too many changes all at once is not a good idea. Not only is it difficult practically, but lots of changes would just build up more autonomic arousal and increase your overload, rather than reduce it.

Imagine trying to cut down on coffee and alcohol the same week as taking up swimming, *and* beginning to eat breakfast! This can seem easy and a novelty for one week, or even two, but then life can quickly get in the way and the new-found lifestyle will quickly slip away.

It is much more effective to make changes one at a time, and to work to some kind of short- and longer-term plan to ensure regular checks on progress. Using your diary at the back of the book can help keep tabs on how you're doing. If you make it part of your new lifestyle to check the diary at a particular time each week, say Sunday night or Monday morning, or whatever, it is much easier to keep going. So, there's no time like the present. Get started!

Finding half an hour to kick a ball about with the family or the neighbours' children a couple of times a week to begin with can be both enjoyable and easy to sustain in the long term. Look for something similar that you can easily fit in, and that you'll actually enjoy and keep doing in the long term. Further changes can then be built on this firm foundation, over a period of time.

So, go back over this list of lifestyle points (pp. 98–100) now, see what you've ticked and make a plan to make a start.

15

Coping with Stress at Work

Today, one of the most common sources of stress, and sometimes unbearable pressure leading to overload, is the workplace. That's pretty well all kinds of workplace – offices, shops, schools, call centres, factories.

Emphasis on job satisfaction has now given way to long hours, down-sizing, short-term contracts, new methods of working, high-pressure call centres, and constant change, which taken together have brought about a sea change in working life in Britain today.

In newspapers and magazines, you'll find many lists of high-stress and low-stress jobs, and your job may be one of the most stressful. But it isn't quite as simple as that. You may have a 'low-stress' job, but may be being bullied by a colleague or manager. Also, no matter what the job is, if it doesn't match your personality, you will feel stressed by it. The outgoing person, who thrives on new activities and meeting new people, would probably find work as a laboratory technician or truck driver hard to cope with. The shrinking violet would probably find life as a double-glazing salesperson or actor difficult.

Causes of workplace stress

Other causes of stress at work are many and varied. The most commonly cited include tight deadlines, constant monitoring, poor internal communications, bullying and excessive hours. A checklist of possible sources follows. You may find much to identify with here – tick or highlight any which apply to you:

Conditions of the job

  uncertainty and insecurity
  poor status, low pay, no promotion prospects
  long or unsociable hours
  shift work, upsetting body's natural rhythms
  insufficient back-up
  unnecessary procedures

travel to and from work (cramped unpunctual trains, long journey, city driving, etc.)
working from home
taking work home
overwork or underwork
time pressure, especially if prolonged
lack of variety
demands made on private and social life
doing job below level of competence
attending meetings
constant monitoring or supervision
amount of travelling
ease of contact – e-mail, fax, bleepers, car phones, mobile phones
  – even at home

Your employer

organizational problems
your beliefs conflicting with your employer's
staff shortages

The job itself

unclear role
role conflict
powerlessness or feeling trapped
unrealistic deadlines
inability to get a job finished
difficult clients or patients
incompetent colleagues
insufficient training
emotional involvement with clients
the responsibilities of it
inability to help or to act effectively
keeping up with new developments or new technology
having to move home often

The job environment

noisy or cramped conditions
excessive heat or humidity
presence of toxic or dangerous materials

Your superiors

clashing with superiors
inadequate leadership

Your subordinates

inadequate training
clashes or difficulties with
having to tell them off

Communication with others

isolation
poor communication or none
conflict with colleagues
unnecessary battles
bullying
discrimination

Your personality and expectations

perfectionist
low tolerance for stress
intolerant of certain behaviours in others, e.g. tidiness,
    punctuality.
competitive personality
lack of confidence
not assertive – either too passive or too aggressive

Problems particularly affecting women

dual role of career and home or family
first woman in the job
having to travel or stay in hotels alone
being conspicuously different
sexism and sexual harassment
male colleagues can feel threatened
promotion can be difficult

In the UK in 2002, one in five people reported having been exposed to high levels of stress at work. Bill Callaghan, Chairperson of the Health and Safety Commission, says that around half a million people in the UK report that they have experienced work-related stress, anxiety or depression at a level that has made them ill. This means 6.5 million working days are lost every year.

But what do you do if you are stressed at work? Workplace stress is just the same as any other stress; basic stress management techniques should be considered, and those which are most relevant should be selected for use. However, the employer probably bears the major responsibility for stress in their workforce, and many organizations are now beginning to take this on board, with many providing helplines or stress workshops.

Think first!

First, it cannot be emphasized enough that great care and thought must be taken before you decide to tackle any problem head-on at work. Suddenly trying out new assertiveness skills on your line manager can endanger a job, and even just admitting to stress can risk a current job or future prospects. So think carefully first, and consider all the options and implications before taking any action.

Tackling the situation

You can tackle this from two different directions.

1 Changing how you think about the situation. Your thinking can be the source of the problem in the first place. It may also be making a minor stress, which can be coped with, into a major one which cannot. So, using the checklist, you should decide whether your thinking has any bearing on each item causing stress. We've already looked at the ways that our thinking can affect us – look back at that chapter now if you need to refresh your memory.

So go back now to the list of causes of stress at work, and put a cross at any cause you've ticked which your thinking may be making a contribution to. Now jot down beside each how you might change your thinking to help you to cope better.

You should then begin working on changing your thinking to reduce the distress slowly but surely. But you should also move on to consider the next area, and how you might resolve the cause of the stress.

2 Resolving the cause of the stress. The next thing you should consider is the overall picture of your workplace stress, and think through these three steps:

Step 1 Are you a square peg in a round hole? Is your personality really not suited to the job? If so, and you can change the job, problem solved. If there is a mis-match, but you can't change the job, you should concentrate on cushioning.

Step 2 Do you have a low tolerance for stress? If so, can you find a less stressful job? If you can't, cushioning is again the best solution.

Step 3 Using the checklist, for each item you've ticked, you should decide whether and how each cause of stress might be resolved. Are you assertive enough? Do you lack other skills? Is there some kind of support system at work? Are you being bullied? Is there support for this? Will trying to do something about the problem put the job or your future at risk? You should also decide whether any of the following would make a difference, and, if so, decide whether to find out more about them:

- assertiveness
- confidence-building
- time management
- delegation
- taking breaks
- learning more about new skills and new technology
- counselling at work
- support for bullying or harassment at work (or outside of work).

So again, go back and jot down against each item ticked anything you feel that could be done to resolve that particular cause.

Cushioning

If having worked through the list of causes of workplace stress, either nothing can be done, or you choose to do nothing, then cushioning is the best option. Cushioning is usually helpful anyway.

   Some employers already provide a range of training, support

systems, employee-assistance programmes, or counselling, and many others are thinking about it. This provision is likely to expand, particularly in the wake of the recent cases of employees having successfully sued their employers for damages due to stress at work, and changes in legislation. If, however, you decide it is prudent to take no direct action on your work stress, the only answer is to cushion yourself from its effects.

Cushioning or dampening the effects of work stress is often the only solution if the way of thinking about the situation cannot be changed, or nothing can be done to change the situation itself. Use all the techniques you've learned in this book to build up your 'resilience' to stress. Looking at your 'work–life balance' is also particularly relevant here, as we've seen when we talked about your lifestyle.

Stress at work is becoming the unchangeable reality for many of us today, and no magic wand seems to be big enough or powerful enough to change that. So putting everything into cushioning yourself so that you can cope better with it is the next best option until circumstances change, as they undoubtedly will some time in the future.

Conclusion: First Aid Summary and Diary

To conclude, here's a summary of immediate 'first aid' you can give yourself whenever you want to rescue yourself from your overload. For easy access, we've summarized this as ten practical tips.

1 Can you do anything about the cause of your autonomic overload?

You may now have some idea of what is causing your autonomic overload, and your first step is to decide whether you can actually do something about this cause:

If you think you can, perhaps you need to seek out expert advice or support on how to deal with the problem. But, one way or another, sort it out. Follow the other nine tips to help you cope while you do this.

If you're sure you can't, do all you can to cushion yourself from its effects, using the rest of this summary to tell you how.

If you're not sure, it may well be that the cause of your autonomic overload is being caused by your lifestyle or general approach to life, and the tips which follow may help sort this out. If you're still not sure, seek out expert advice and support to help clarify the situation.

2 Slow down and make time for relaxation

There are all sorts of ways to relax. The important thing is that you allow your body to slow down and completely relax at least once every day: a lazy bath, a walk, a visit to friends, music, yoga, sport, and so on. Relaxation exercises are useful because you can usually fit them into your day, and they can also help keep autonomic overload under control in problem situations. With practice, you should be able to relax in just a few minutes, or even less.

Begin by practising the methods given in this book every day, until they begin to work for you. Then you can use them as a regular relaxing break, and to help you to cope better with those difficult situations.

It is sometimes useful to join a relaxation group in your area, especially if it's hard to get the time and space at home. Yoga classes are another option as they usually end with a relaxation session.

If your time is tight, you may think that taking time to do this will just get you even further behind, but this is not the case. If your body is allowed to relax regularly, you will be able to get more done more effectively with the time left, because you are refreshed and energized.

You can also relax your mind as follows:

- Slow down and relax your body.
- Once relaxed, picture as clearly as you can, or focus your mind on any one of these:
    waves lapping on the sea-shore;
    branches swaying in the breeze;
    deep, dark green velvet;
    a word or phrase such as 'peace', 'calm', 'relax';
    a calming poem, prayer or picture.

3 Think about your breathing

Breathing normally can help to relieve many of the symptoms of autonomic overload, and will also help you cope better in difficult situations. Breathing techniques are also an alternative way to relax. Here is a simple technique to help you to slow and regulate your breathing, yet still remain alert.

- Lie or sit with good support.
- Let your breath go, then take a gentle breath in to your own slow silent count of 1 . . . . 2 . . . . 3. Then breathe out in your own time, again to your own slow and silent count of 1 . . . . 2 . . . . 3.
- Continue gently breathing to this rhythm for a few minutes.

With practice, you will be able to leave out the counting, and just go into this rhythm when you need to.

4 Take regular breaks

Managing your time is key. Taking regular breaks, especially from a difficult situation, will leave you refreshed and able to cope better and work more efficiently on your return; even a five-minute break in a tiring morning can work wonders. Remember to make time for yourself, and for hobbies, interests and leisure pursuits; this takes your mind off your troubles, and helps to keep them in perspective. Conversely, if you have too much time on your hands, get involved in a hobby or voluntary activity, preferably with other people. Whatever your situation, ensure you do things you enjoy regularly.

If time is tight:

- keep lists of jobs to be done, separating urgent and non-urgent;
- select and prioritize what you do – you can't do it all;
- plan your days and weeks in advance and keep a diary;
- be organized and know where everything is;
- do one job at a time;
- delegate whenever possible.

5 Adopt a 'cushioning' lifestyle

Here are some general tips. Remember to tick or highlight those you think apply to you, and make changes one at a time, with your progress diary to help you keep track.

General

- Eat a well-balanced diet, low in sugar, salt and fat, and high in fibre.
- Don't skip meals, especially breakfast and lunch.
- Avoid food or drink containing caffeine, e.g. cola, coffee, chocolate.
- Do not use alcohol or other substances to help you sleep or relax.
- Bear in mind the recommended weekly alcohol intake if you do drink.
- Get plenty of restful sleep – use relaxation or breathing if you can't get off to sleep, or you wake up during the night.

Exercise

- Regular physical activity that you enjoy and that fits in with your lifestyle is a very good cushion for autonomic overload.
- Walking is generally all right for most people, but if you're unsure about beginning or resuming a particular form of exercise, check with your doctor first.

- A contact sport is particularly useful if you are suppressing anger or frustration due to work or some other situation.

6 Coping with panic attacks

The key is to catch them early, and stop them in their tracks. This puts you back in control. Here is one way of doing this. Don't be put off if this method doesn't work the first or even second time you try it. Keep at it; it can be very effective:

Work out what are your own first signs of a panic attack. This might be a lurch in the stomach, a thought in your mind, heart rate rising, or something else you've noticed.

Look out for these first signs, and when you notice them you should immediately PAUSE:

- **P**ause ... and make yourself comfortable (sit down, lean on something etc.).
- **A**bsorb ... detail of what's going on around you.
- **U**se ... any method of relaxing quickly which works well for you, then
- **S**lowly ... when you feel better,
- **E**ase ... yourself back into what you were doing.

7 Watch out for your thinking style

Your thinking may contribute to your autonomic overload, and being aware of this can make a real difference. We all know people who seem to cope with anything. The difference is usually in their attitude to life. Here are some ideas to think about. Tick or highlight anything which might apply to you.

- Avoid negative thinking. Acknowledge the bad side of life, but don't dwell on it.
- Don't ignore the ordinary or good things that happen each day as if they don't count for some reason.
- Bear in mind that when things go wrong it's not always your fault. Other people or simply the situation are just as often to blame.
- Take your mind off your problems as much as you can. They grow bigger the more you concentrate on them.

- Avoid 'should', 'ought' and 'must' thinking. Do you often find yourself using one of these words, 'I must do this', 'I ought to do that', and so on? Ask yourself who is setting these personal standards and targets, and whether you are setting them too high.
- Change mistaken beliefs. Your whole thinking may have at its heart one or more mistaken assumptions, such as, 'I'm a failure if I make a mistake', 'I should be happy/successful all the time', 'People must always like me', or, 'Life should be fair'.

8 Hone your assertiveness skills

Assertiveness is often wrongly confused with being aggressive and self-centred. This could hardly be further from the truth. Assertiveness is about having respect for yourself and others, knowing and expressing your needs, and being able to compromise with others.

If a lot of what we do is not assertive, this can cause autonomic overload. When we are not assertive we are likely to be either manipulative, aggressive or passively giving in to others.

A main factor in assertiveness is learning to refuse unwelcome suggestions or tasks.

- Feel free to say no;
- keep it short, and say it confidently and warmly;
- only give a reason if you want to;
- use a simple phrase you're comfortable with, such as 'I don't want to', or 'I'd rather not';
- calmly repeat your 'No' if the first one is not accepted.

Remember you have these rights:
- to make a mistake
- to have your own point of view
- to fail if you try something
- to try again
- to expect others to listen to you.

Deal with your anger when you're alone by:
- punching a pillow, cushion, bed – anything soft that you won't damage
- tearing up old newspapers

- writing down your angry feelings, then tearing them up!

Other assertiveness tips:

- value yourself
- value other people
- work out what you need and want out of life
- be prepared to compromise
- keep to any point you're making – don't let others distract you from it
- keep your voice slow, steady and low-pitched, and stay relaxed
- get your feeling of self-worth from within yourself, not just from other people.

9 A problem shared . . .

We all need someone who cares about us and what we do. Be careful only to confide in those you can trust, whether it's family, friends, partner, colleagues, or confidential support groups or others in your community. It is no sign of weakness to seek such support. It can be really effective, and it is a strength to recognize this.

10 Check your work-related overload

Cushion yourself from work-related overload by using the tips covered so far, especially relaxation, breaks, social support, a healthy lifestyle, and leisure activities. Think very carefully before you tackle a problem head-on at work. Remember there may be repercussions for your job or future career.

Here are some other general pointers to think about:

- Are you a square peg in a round hole? Does your personality not really suit the job? If so, and you can change your job, this may be a solution. If you can't, cushioning is the best answer.
- Perhaps you have a low tolerance for autonomic overload. Many people do. If so, can you find a less demanding job? If not, cushioning is again the best solution.
- Would learning some new skills make a difference? What about assertiveness, confidence-building, time management, team-working, delegation, new technology? Are courses like this available to you either at work or from adult education?

- Is confidential counselling available at work? Some employers now provide this entirely separately and independent of the workplace.

Main points

- Can you do anything about the cause?
- Slow down and relax every day.
- Make sure you are breathing normally.
- Take breaks regularly.
- Adopt a lifestyle which cushions you – regular healthy meals, lots of sleep, exercise, leisure.
- Get control of the panic attacks.
- Watch out for your thinking causing autonomic overload.
- Become more assertive if you need to.
- Share your troubles.
- Think about how you can best tackle autonomic overload at work.

Remember

This is a problem only you can solve. You may need assistance, and informed help is always useful and welcome, but in the final analysis it is your commitment and determination that will bring the rewards. You can do it. If you really want to, you will do it. It's up to you.

Good luck!

Progress Diary

At the end of each week, keep a note here of your own rating of how autonomic overloaded you are on a scale of 0 (no problem) to 5 (maximum problem). Jot down any actions you've decided to take, progress on previous new tactics tried, and so on.

Progress diary

Date	Autonomic overload rating (0 min – 5 max)	Actions planned/Progress on previous actions

CONCLUSION: FIRST AID AND DIARY

Date	Autonomic overload rating (0 min – 5 max)	Actions planned/Progress on previous actions

Useful Resources

Here are some useful addresses of national organizations (many have local contacts or groups, or have distance-learning courses or support available).

Alice Muir Life Coaching
Mains of Lochridge
Stewarton
Kilmarnock
Ayrshire KA3 5LH
Tel: 01560 486888
E-mail: stresscourses@lineone.net
Website: www.stress-confidence.com

Association for Post Natal Illness
145 Dawes Road
Fulham
London SW6 7EB
Helpline: 020 7386 0868
E-mail: info@apni.org
Website: www.apni.org

British Association for Counselling and Psychotherapy
BACP House
35–37 Albert Street
Rugby
Warwickshire CV21 2SG
Tel: 0870 443 5252
E-mail: bacp@bacp.co.uk
Website: www.bacp.co.uk

Child Bereavement Trust
Aston House
West Wycombe
High Wycombe
Bucks HP14 3AG
Tel: 0845 357 1000
E-mail: enquiries@childbereavement.org.uk
Website: www.childbereavement.org.uk

Childline 0800 1111
Cruse Bereavement Care
126 Sheen Road
Richmond
Surrey TW9 1UR
Helpline: 0870 167 1677
E-mail: helpline@crusebereavementcare.org.uk
Website: www.crusebereavementcare.org.uk

Depression Alliance
212 Spitfire Studios
63–71 Collier Street
London N1 9BE
Helpline: 0845 123 23 20
E-mail: information@depressionalliance.org
Website: www.depressionalliance.org

Drinkline 0800 917 8282

Health and Safety Executive Information Services
Caerphilly Park
Caerphilly CF83 3GG
HSE Infoline 0845 345 0055
Website: www.hse.gov.uk
Provides up-to-date books, press releases, leaflets, etc. and resources to download free

International Stress Management Association UK
PO Box 26
South Petherton
Somerset TA13 5WY
Tel: 07000 780430
E-mail: stress@isma.org.uk
Website: www.isma.org.uk

Mind Publications
15–19 Broadway
London E15 4BQ
Mindinfoline: 0845 766 0163
E-mail: contact@mind.org.uk
Website: www.mind.org.uk
Full catalogue of useful books, leaflets and order form available

National Association for Premenstrual Syndrome
41 Old Road
East Peckham
Kent TN12 5AP
Helpline: 0870 777 2177
E-mail: contact@pms.org.uk
Website: www.pms.org.uk

National Drugs Helpline 0800 776600
Website: www.urban75.com/drugs

No Panic
93 Brands Farm Way
Randlay
Telford
Shropshire TF3 2JQ
Helpline: 0808 808 0545
E-mail: ceo@nopanic.org.uk
Website: www.nopanic.org.uk

Parentline Plus Helpline 0808 800 2222

Relate (National Marriage Guidance)
Herbert Gray College
Little Church Street
Rugby
Warwickshire CV21 3AP
Helpline: 0845 456 1310
Website: www.relate.org.uk

Relaxation for Living Trust
168–170 Oatlands Drive
Weybridge
Surrey KT13 9ET
Produces cassettes, leaflets, etc.

Samaritans
National Helpline 08457 90 90 90
Or see local telephone directory

Scottish Association for Mental Health
Cumbrae House
15 Carlton Court
Glasgow G5 9JP
Tel: 0141 568 7000
E-mail: enquire@samh.org.uk
Website: www.samh.org.uk

Stillbirth and Neonatal Death Society
28 Portland Place
London W1B 1LY
Helpline: 020 7436 5881
E-mail: helpline@uk-sands.org
Website: www.uk-sands.org

Stress Education Services
Mains of Lochridge
Stewarton
Kilmarnock
Ayrshire KA3 5LH
Tel: 01560 486888
E-mail: stresscourses@lineone.net
Website: www.stresstrain.co.uk
Provides CDs, distance-learning courses and coaching

Turning Point
New Loom House
101 Backchurch Lane
London E1 1LU
Helpline: 020 7702 2300
E-mail: info@turning-point.co.uk
Website: www.turning-point.co.uk

Victim Support
Cranmer House
39 Brixton Road
London SW9 6DZ
Tel: 020 7735 9166
Website www.victimsupport.org

Women's Aid Federation
PO Box 391
Bristol BS99 7WS
Helpline: 0845 7023468

Workplace Bullying Advice Line 01235 212286

Index